Finding your Well-*BEing*

The path to happiness, clarity and peace

Mary Mangos

First published 2021 by Mary Mangos

Produced by Indie Experts P/L, Australasia
indieexperts.com.au

Copyright © Mary Mangos 2021

The moral right of the author to be identified as the author of this work has been asserted.

Except for the purposes of reviewing, no part of this publication may be reproduced or transmitted in any form or by any means, electronic or mechanical, including photocopying, recording or any information storage or retrieval system, without the written permission of the author. Infringers of copyright render themselves viable for prosecution.

Cover design by Daniela Catucci @ Catucci Design
Edited by Anne-Marie Tripp @ Indie Experts
Internal design by Indie Experts
Typeset in 11/16 pt Kepler Std by Post Pre-press Group, Brisbane

ISBN 978-0-6452613-0-1 (paperback)
ISBN 978-0-6452613-1-8 (epub)

Disclaimer: Every effort has been made to ensure this book is as accurate and complete as possible. However, there may be mistakes both typographical and in content. Therefore, this book should be used as a general guide and is not the ultimate source of information contained herein. The author and publisher shall not be liable or responsible to any person or entity with respect to any loss or damage caused or alleged to have been caused directly or indirectly by the information contained in this book.

Contents

Foreword — vii

Introduction: My Well-*BEing* Mission — 1
Chapter 1: The State of Our Wellbeing — 11
Chapter 2: Find Your Energy Zen — 29
Chapter 3: Cultivating Mindful Clarity — 43
Chapter 4: Happiness Through Gratitude — 65
Chapter 5: The Power of Affirmations and
 Positive Self-Talk — 83
Chapter 6: Spirituality for Wisdom and Peace — 101
Chapter 7: Your Self-Care Plan — 119
Chapter 8: Final Thoughts for Your Journey — 139

Acknowledgements — 143
About Mary Mangos — 147
Work with Mary Mangos — 149
Notes — 151
Bibliography — 157

Dear reader

As a bonus, I wish to give you a FREE gift to support your journey towards wellbeing and well-*BEing*. I have created a *Finding Your Well-BEing Workbook* for you to use as you work through this book. It will provide a guide to your wellbeing journey, the tools to support your practice, and the space to record your reflections.

Download the free *Finding Your Well-BEing Workbook* at the Coachuwellness website, at:
https://www.coachuwellness.com.au/downloads

Foreword

'Resilience is More Than a Mindset', an episode of *Wellness Solutions* with Mary Mangos, was the very first podcast I participated in as the author of the *Multi-System Model of Resilience (https://msmrtool.com)*. During this podcast, it was clear that Mary and I shared a passion and excitement to create awareness about mental health. We want to share with the world that mental health is not about telling someone what the right or wrong things are to do. Instead, it's about honouring each person's respective journey and processes.

As a health psychologist, educator, and researcher, I am dedicating my career to the study of resilience. How do we find resilience, when do we use resilience, and how does resilience inform our wellbeing? I am excited by Mary's book *Finding Your Well-BEing*. This book connects us through shared goals and struggles. Importantly, it transforms the science of wellbeing into real-life. In these pages, science becomes practice, and practice becomes reality.

Discovering our mental health often begins with steps taken to reflect on our challenges. Through personal accounts and candid stories from her past, Mary takes us on her path to discovering her wellbeing. Mary weaves research, tools, and tips across diverse sub-fields of positive psychology along with her unique insights as a practitioner and mental health expert. Readers are introduced to both the science of wellbeing, and ways to integrate them into everyday activities.

Being well while your world is crumbling, your children crying, and you've got back-to-back meetings in the calendar can seem downright impossible. What is this elusive wellbeing we seem to be perpetually seeking? What are the factors that make us well? Through this book, you learn how to be well by simply *BE*ing – the best versions of yourselves!

Mary's book is an honest journey on becoming a better you. And it is something we can all relate to and learn from.

Dr Jenny Liu
Author, *Multi-System Model of Resilience*
Postdoctoral Associate & Adjunct Research Professor
Department of Psychiatry, Schulich School of Medicine, Western University

Wellbeing is not just being healthy and avoiding illness, it is a complex combination of physical, mental, emotional and social factors that lead to a happy and satisfying life.

Well-*BEing* is about your active, present, ongoing engagement in behaviours and choices that promote wellbeing and allow you to *be* your best. Well-*BEing* is something that you *do*, and places the emphasis on *being* right now, in the moment, not worrying about the past or the future.

INTRODUCTION
My Well-*BEing* Mission

> 'As for the future, it remains unwritten. Anything can happen, and often we are wrong. The best we can do with the future is to prepare and savour the possibilities of what can be done in the present.'
>
> **Todd Kashdan**

I have a mission, a dream and hope, to inspire you to change your life toward more happiness, clarity and peace. I have had many opportunities to reflect and reaffirm my mission over the last 18 months as I navigated the COVID-19 lockdowns. I found it more challenging to manage the uncertainty, create new routines and deal with my increasing stress and fatigue. I have more appreciation of my strengths and abilities. I am proud of the decisions I am making to prioritise my needs, my wellbeing. It has also reinforced my purpose to make a positive difference to *your* wellbeing.

The fourth lockdown of Melbourne, Australia, in June 2021 was one of the most impactful for many people, including myself. The president of the Australian Psychological Society, Tamara Cavenett, suggested that this lockdown was worse for many as a result of the extended period of worry leading into it, and the compounding fatigue of previous lockdowns.[1] And now as I write this, the two most populated states in Australia are yet again in lockdown – making this our fifth lockdown in Melbourne – after being affected by the highly contagious Delta strain of the virus. If I thought lockdown number four was bad, well, lockdown number five has taken it to another level. I made the decision to prioritise my health and stop working on my book during the first week of this current lockdown. I reduced my priorities to deal with an onset of more fatigue. It has been another great reminder for me that nothing is more important than our well-*BEing*.

Before I explain what I mean by 'well-*BEing*', it's important to first explain what 'wellness' and 'wellbeing' are, and how they relate to each other. Wellness refers to our physical health. It is not only the freedom from illness or bad health, but it also involves engaging in practices that lead to positive health outcomes, including the prevention of disability or disease.[2]

Wellness is part of wellbeing, but wellbeing is a much broader concept; 'a complex combination of a person's physical, mental, emotional and social health factors.'[3] It involves cultivating and experiencing happiness and life satisfaction. Aspects of our lives that have a positive impact on our wellbeing include close and happy relationships with partners and friends; a nutritious diet and regular exercise; the ability to adapt to change and uncertainty; good self-esteem and a positive outlook; and spiritual or religious beliefs.[4]

When I refer to 'well-*BEing*', I'm building on this definition even further. I believe there is nothing more important than to experience wellbeing, prioritising yourself, your life, and your happiness. But when you emphasise and focus on '*BEing*', you are actively living in the moment, not worrying about the past or the future. Instead, you are liv*ing* well, right now, in the present. Well-*BEing* is something that you do. It is about your behaviours, actions, choices and the outcome of your commitments and priorities that promote your wellbeing. It involves identifying what is important to you, what you care about and how you spend your time to shape a life lived well. As Socrates once said:

'To BE is to DO.'

My passion for wellbeing, and well-*BEing*, has been important to me over a long period. My mission, my dream and my hope has unfolded and become a clearer priority for me personally, as I navigated life's challenges towards my personal wellbeing goals. I grew up in a family environment where I experienced joy and love. I was encouraged to keep a strong faith and appreciate opportunities, but at the same time have an awareness that things could change for the worse at any moment. I remember being around seven years of age, sitting with my family over dinner and my dad starting a discussion about how, as immigrants, our position in this country was not certain. He talked about how we needed to be mentally prepared because one day we might be sent back to Greece.

This fear my dad shared with us was not necessarily based on the reality of where we lived in Australia, but rather what he felt was happening in Europe. In addition, my dad, as an Australian citizen, was appreciative of our opportunities whilst being very fearful that things could change. I know that my beautiful parents were trying to protect us from what they believed were very real, possible negative life events, but his fear was contagious. It taught me to worry about the future and to be on alert. To be able to look at potential issues and problems can be a wonderful capability, but in my case, it shaped a strongly pessimistic view of the world.

This perspective of how I saw my life continued through my adulthood and even during my psychology studies at university. As a young adult, I would often not cope well with stressors and adversities. One vivid memory I have is during my fifth year of university studies, getting my first migraine that required hospitalisation, while I was writing my thesis. I was working long hours, I had lost any perspective around the need for life balance, and at that stage of my life, I did not value the importance of rest and energy management.

It took me weeks to recover and get back to what I thought was a 'normal healthy state' to return to my university studies. Being forced to do nothing but rest did give me some time to reflect. I began to develop a holistic view of what contributed to my wellness. I explored yoga and meditation, and tried acupuncture and reiki as I questioned what best supported me. I was searching for practices to make me feel better. At this stage of my life, it was a short-term fix that I was after, not a change to my life.

It was during my 30s that I became exposed to the science and research of *positive psychology*. I learnt that we should and could expect more from our lives and how we felt. I learnt that it was possible to cultivate practices that supported a thriving life. My enthusiasm and renewed inspiration took a major positive turn when I read my first positive psychology book – *Learned Optimism: How to Change Your Mind and Your Life* by Professor Martin Seligman, a pioneer of positive psychology. I was in my mid 30s and I had a significant revelation when I read this book. It revealed to me that I am strongly pessimistic, even though I approached the world with a smile and positivity through my behaviour and actions. I learnt that my pessimistic tendencies meant that I would most likely interpret situations or problems in a negative way: focusing on all the negatives, what could go wrong, what should have happened, and the risks in the future. This approach affected my enjoyment of the present.

I also learnt that I could shift that pessimism. This helped me to develop more clarity around what my life could become. With practice and discipline, I could lean towards some great practices that could build my hope, optimism and cultivate a sense of calm. I did not need to live like this anymore. I could choose to have a life that was more joyful, more inspiring; a life where I was present and in the moment. It took some years to hone those practices and I have always loved sharing them with clients and seeing *their* results.

In my 40s, I began to explore mindfulness research and programs. I undertook professional development to learn stress-reduction mindfulness-meditation techniques. I began to think about how to integrate some of these practices into my daily life. My reflections commenced with an exploration of what was stopping me integrating practices that I knew were helpful. Meditation, for example, I found to be challenging. Sitting in stillness for long periods felt stressful and painful. I wondered if trying shorter meditations would help overcome this blocker for me. At the time there were not many resources with shorter guided meditation practices that included music. I decided to solve this problem by creating my own. I added music to soothe my negative feelings and to induce feelings of calm.

I then explored and experimented with how to make meditation part of my normal routine. What worked well for me, I discovered, was to approach my practice with flexibility and self-compassion. If I missed a day or if I did not want to meditate, or if I wanted to mediate only for a few minutes, I told myself 'well done', or 'a few minutes is better than no minutes', or 'there is always tomorrow'. This flexibility and compassion with how I approach implementing positive practices is essential to how I integrate it successfully into my life.

My hope is to provide you with inspiration, comfort and a practical way forward. I hope that you can feel hope in the power of making positive change in your life, other lives and your communities. The good news is that it *is* in your power, and we often call this power your *agency*. According to Professor Albert Bandura, *agency* 'refers to the human capability to influence one's functioning and the course of events by one's actions.'[5] It involves:

- forming intentions, plans and strategies

- having forethought to visualise the future, set goals, consider blockers and your motivation
- taking action, monitoring progress and self-correcting
- self-reflection on your values, goals to make the best choices for you.

Having a sense of agency that can influence your thoughts and behaviours is important. It will influence your ability to stay flexible and resilient in the face of adversity and change. You may feel you have very little agency in your lifes; that things happen and how you respond is something that simply *is what it is*. I encourage you to open the door to the possibility of being able to influence your life, your thinking and your behaviours.

The ideas and strategies in this book have a core foundational belief: *Even during real human challenges, you can lead a happier life.* A life where you feel you are thriving. A life where you take care of your mind, body, emotions and spirit. This can be a life where you still feel pain, frustration and sadness, but a life where you can take your power back through your agency.

Let's break through the complexity, by focusing on your intentions and cultivating peace. This will create more clarity to live your best life and thrive, and to explore your priorities and the practices that matter to you.

This book will explore ideas to help you to go beyond improving your wellness, and support your agency to achieve your wellbeing vision and goals. It is designed to enhance your well-*BEing* so that you feel you are living your best life. To feel that you are well by leaning into what is in your control. You can control your inner thoughts, your feelings, your narrative and your compassion. You will be encouraged towards actions that you can take to prepare, reflect, implement and influence how you experience your life. I will step you through the state of our wellbeing (chapter 1), to understand where wellbeing is at today and what impact the COVID-19 pandemic is having. You will explore what supports your energy and how to renew your energy zen (chapter 2).

I will share information and strategies that can help you to cultivate your mindful clarity (chapter 3); becoming more aware of when you are on autopilot, setting your intention, learning how to embrace uncertainty, welcoming all emotions and how to move towards peace and joy.

I will help you to consider how gratitude can create a life for you that is happier and supports your resilience, so that you can persevere through tough times (chapter 4). Using the power of affirmations and positive self-talk (chapter 5), I will show you how to prepare your mindset for positive actions and behaviours that work towards the life that you most desire.

I outline my own spiritual journey (chapter 6), pivotal life events and practices that supported me towards wisdom and peace; these may help you, too. In this chapter and throughout the book, I share real human experiences, including my own, to inspire your journey towards wellness.

Lastly, I will explain to you how to create your self-care plan (chapter 7). This will include how to identify your vision, the practices you will focus on and learning how to integrate them. You will learn how to make your practices sustainable so that you continue your well-*BEing* path over the long term.

Throughout the book, I will be encouraging you to actively participate and create a journey that best suits you. You will regularly stop, reflect and complete some practices. There is space to record your answers in this book; alternatively, download the FREE *Finding Your Well-BEing Workbook* from https://coachuwellness.com.au/downloads. This workbook has been created as a gift to support your wellbeing journey. It will provide a guide to your wellbeing journey, the tools to support your practice and extra space to record your reflections.

Please be kind to yourself. Take self-compassion seriously and go at your own pace. Trust your intuition and explore what feels important to you right now. Whether you work through all of the chapters in order or just immerse yourself in the ideas of one chapter, that is amazing. **One small change to your wellbeing can make a huge difference.**

For many years I was languishing and at times my mental health also declined, and I was diagnosed with depression. I have had poor emotional and mental health, which impacted my work, my relationships and my physical energy. I dedicate my book to that young woman I once was and I want to give her hope, love and direction. Things can be different. Life can be better.

My wish for YOU is to discover that internal inspiration, to carve out some time and explore how to focus on YOURSELF during these challenging times. Let this book support you to make the positive changes you deserve. I hope it inspires you to shape your well-*BEing*, and to live your life with purpose and thrive.

CHAPTER 1
The State of Our Wellbeing

'Even in the worst times, joy and happiness are possible.'
Dr Maria Sirois

I want to share with you the current state of our wellbeing and happiness; how the COVID-19 pandemic has impacted us; what stress is and how it affects us. Let me begin by sharing **my state of wellbeing**. In the introduction, I shared my mission to inspire you to change your life toward more happiness, clarity and peace. For me, I have found the ebb and flow of my emotions during the COVID-19 pandemic has sometimes felt like a rollercoaster – and I don't like rollercoasters!

At the beginning of the pandemic, I remember watching the news coverage one night, gripping my glass of wine so tightly, and feeling waves of uncertainty and stress wash over me. During those early days in particular, my sleep, my mood and my productivity were affected. I would wake up feeling tired. I was checking in constantly with family members to make sure they were okay. I listened to their fears and concerns. I began to feel increasingly impacted by their distress, as my stress response was already activated. Professionally, everything seemed to take longer to get done. I soon recognised that while this was a normal response, it was far from ideal. The pandemic's impact was preventing me from communicating effectively and was affecting my wellbeing on many levels. I had to re-assess my self-care practices and avoid numbing myself with alcohol to cope with my stress and fear.

My friends and clients were contacting me, looking for resources and programs that they could access for themselves or to provide their staff. People were looking for how to better process what was happening and move forward. It was abundantly clear to me that I needed to revisit my own self-care to refocus my sense of agency, if I was going to quickly create these programs and support others effectively. I decided to focus on the following changes to my self-care practices:

- more meditation
- more breaks whilst working
- exercising regularly
- better nutrition
- ensuring my news exposure was limited.

Like many of you, I stayed connected with loved ones virtually to overcome loneliness and to bring more joy into my life. I challenged myself to channel my fear into a strong sense of purpose to ensure others had strategies to process this experience, renew themselves and move towards a more flourishing mental and emotional space.

What I underestimated was the extent to which this world experience and my workload would fatigue me. Feeling the pain, frustration and uncertainty that others shared, and focusing on serving as many people as I could, negatively impacted my wellbeing. Whilst I took breaks consistently during the day, I didn't consider taking more regular holiday breaks. I associated staying at home with working. Unfortunately, I got to Christmas 2020 and I felt depleted and fatigued.

The first few months of 2021 were a journey of re-assessing my self-care practices and making the necessary positive changes I needed. I also sought professional advice, seeing my integrative medicine general practitioner and talking to my psychology supervisor to ensure I took a holistic approach and stayed on course with my plan. I encourage you to do the same, and seek advice from a trusted professional if you feel fatigued, too.

I have learnt to prioritise myself first again; even though I'm not sure I was ever that great at doing this. If I reflect back on myself as a young adult, I remember how I wanted to always be there for my children and so I would sacrifice many of my personal wellbeing goals. I didn't want to miss anything or to not measure up to the unrealistic ideal of what makes a great parent. I know many of you will relate to the experience of prioritising your children, often before yourself. What we learn with time and reflection is that our lives and parenting skills may have been so much better with some attention to ourselves. Whilst we can't go back and change the past, we can make a difference to the present and our future. It is not too late to prioritise yourself NOW.

To find more moments of peace and zen has been life changing. I took a few weeks away early this year (2021) from work to renew my energy, and focus on actively cultivating practices that helped me to feel well *now*; practices that support my well-*BEing*. I am committed to taking more days and more weeks for myself over the next few months and years. I know this is very important in a world full of uncertainty as a result of the COVID-19 pandemic. I am very mindful of my mental health and wellbeing and I have the clarity and commitment to give it the attention it deserves.

Pandemic Impact

The 2021 *World Happiness Report* highlights how mental health has been a key component to our wellbeing as we experience this pandemic, and notes that mental health:

> 'is also a risk factor for future physical health and longevity, which will be a leading indicator of the future, indirect long-run health consequences of the pandemic. Mental health will influence and drive a number of other individual choices, behaviours, and outcomes.'[6]

This report identifies mental health as one part of our wellbeing most significantly impacted by the COVID-19 pandemic and the resulting lockdowns, noting:

- a worsening of mental health in many countries worldwide
- a higher representation of mental health problems among young people, women, those who lost jobs, and those of lower socio-economic status
- a significant disruption of mental healthcare services despite increasing needs for them.

Recent survey data from the United States highlights the pandemic's negative impact on mental health, with nearly one third of Americans now showing signs of clinical levels of depression or anxiety.[7] We have also seen a widespread increase in psychological symptoms here in Australia, including anxiety, depression and irritability.[8]

It is no surprise that the COVID-19 pandemic has been associated with a substantial rise in symptoms of mental ill-health. Lockdowns, restrictions, isolation and profound loss has occurred. Even as vaccination programs get traction, restrictions of varying severity still come and go to manage outbreaks. The uncertainty of when the pandemic will end still continues in our lives and has consequences for our mental health and wellbeing. This is compounding the (pre-pandemic) state of our mental health, where depression was already identified as one of the leading causes of disability by the World Health Organisation, with high individual and community costs:

> 'Mental health conditions can have a substantial effect on all areas of life, such as school or work performance, relationships with family and friends and ability to

participate in the community. Two of the most common mental health conditions, depression and anxiety, cost the global economy US$1 trillion each year.'[9]

In Australia alone, the pre-pandemic cost of mental ill-health to the Australian economy was estimated to be, conservatively, in the order of $70 billion per year, with an additional cost of approximately $150 billion per year associated with diminished health and reduced life expectancy for those living with mental ill-health.[10] These are huge numbers, reflecting real people who are living with the experience of poor mental health or who are caring for others in their families or communities.

The effect of our current circumstances has left many of us feeling challenged, stressed and overwhelmed. Few would disagree that the fallout from the pandemic has been significant, and what is concerning is the potential – and likely – continued impact on our wellbeing.

Learning to live in this environment of uncertainty is now an important priority for us all. Developing our capability to prioritise ourselves and be flexible with our plans to make adjustments that serve us best will go a long way towards positive outcomes. Where do you start? Let's begin by understanding stress and why we are motivated to pursue certainty.

Stress and Uncertainty

You might use the word 'stress' to describe when you feel overwhelmed, tense and worried, or when you feel that you're dealing with a situation that might be threatening or challenging to cope with.[11] Stress is a biological phenomenon which describes the impact of factors in your life or mind on your wellbeing.[12] Stress can occur across many different situations, and can vary in severity and duration. Some of the different types of stress[13] you might experience include:

- **Trauma**, involving significant threats of injury or death. These might be individual, or happen to many people at the same time. Examples of trauma include car accidents, severe interpersonal violence, war, or experiencing natural disasters such as a flood.

- **Life events** such as bereavement or divorce. These are events that happen to individuals, and cause a negative change to that person's environment. Losing your job or having to close your business as a result of the COVID-19 pandemic are examples of stressful life events.

- **Chronic stress**, which can come from chronic illness, unresolved long-term conflicts, ongoing uncertainty, poor working conditions, poverty, or abusive family situations. The experience of constant change and uncertainty as a result of the COVID-19 pandemic is an example of chronic stress that some may experience.

- **Daily stressors**, which are normally minor issues of relatively short duration. Some examples include a challenging conversation with a loved one, a breakdown of your washing machine, or even a new project that increases your workload.

As human beings it is normal for us to strive to reduce our uncertainty.

> 'Our ancestors were motivated to find stable sources of food, water and shelter to survive and protect their families. This deep need for certainty is true today as we work to address our basic needs and provide for ourselves and loved ones in a highly unpredictable world.'[14]

We desire to create certainty about future outcomes through our beliefs about it. If we view our experience of uncertainty with curiosity, our stress response may be moderated. In contrast, we may feel a lot of stress about our experience if we believe we lack control over the situation and what strategy or action to choose. Also, when stressors from trauma, chronic stress, or life events are always present and you feel impacted by them, your stress response may stay activated and may not return to normal.

What Happens When You Feel Stress?

When you experience something that might be dangerous, threatening or worrying, your sense organs (eyes, ears, nose, etc.) send a message to a small structure in the brain called the amygdala. The amygdala plays a big part in processing emotions, memories, and decisions. The amygdala interprets the messages from your senses, and if it does perceive danger, it immediately sends a distress signal to another part of the brain called the hypothalamus.

The hypothalamus is a really important part of your brain, and is largely responsible for maintaining balance in your body, including regulating processes like body temperature, heart rate and blood pressure, thirst and hunger, sleep, and the production of hormones.[15]

When the hypothalamus is activated in a stressful situation, it sends a signal to your adrenal glands to quickly release a surge of hormones into the bloodstream, particularly adrenaline and cortisol.[16] These are the hormones largely responsible for the body's 'fight or flight' response, helping your body channel its resources so you have the energy to either fight or escape from the perceived danger. Adrenaline causes an increase in your heart rate, blood pressure, and breathing rate, and cortisol increases the amount of glucose (sugar) in your bloodstream, which gives a big, immediate boost of energy to your muscles.

Short bursts of adrenaline and cortisol can be useful and energising, preparing you to take action, sharpening your focus and increasing your strength, and temporarily decreasing your sensitivity to pain. It's important to understand that even minor daily stressors can trigger a stress response. A surprising challenge, such as increased workload, may cause you to react to it as a perceived threat. However, if stress becomes prolonged or chronic and your stress response stays activated over a long period of time, the ongoing overexposure to these stress hormones can have significant, negative effects on your physical and mental health.[17]

Some of the consequences from chronic stress may include:

- the reduction of the size of some structures in your brain and less neural plasticity, potentially causing cognitive, emotional and behavioural dysfunctions[18]
- a higher risk of developing neurodegenerative diseases including sporadic Alzheimer's disease[19]
- chronic inflammatory changes that may result in atherosclerosis in the arteries[20]
- diabetes, cancer, autoimmune syndromes and mental illnesses such as depression.[21]

How do you know if stress is impacting you? Consider if you have ever noticed the following symptoms of chronic stress:

Physical symptoms such as heart palpitations, fatigue, sleep disturbance, insomnia, stomach upset, diarrhea, frequent headaches, muscular aches and pains, weakened immune system, high blood pressure.

Psychological symptoms such as worry, fear, anger, tearfulness, irritability, anxiety, helplessness, difficulties with concentration or memory, or feeling overwhelmed."[22]

Put the Brakes on YOUR Stress

The good news is that you can learn HOW to put the *brakes* on stress. You can become more aware of the energy your stress response is putting into your body and how it is impacting you, and you can learn to manage and release it. You can normalise how you view uncertainty, and increase your sense of control and agency to protect and promote your wellbeing. Throughout the chapters that follow you will find inspiring ideas to consider and explore that will support you. These ideas and the content shared are aligned with many of the key protective factors important for happiness and wellbeing outlined in the recent *World Happiness Report*[23] *including:*

- gratitude – noticing your blessings and express appreciation[24]
- resilience – your ability to recover from adversity, your mindset, and your community and social resources that you rely on get back to coping or thriving[25]
- grit – being able to maintain effort despite failure, stress or adversity[26]
- flow – when you feel immersed, happy and in control of activities[27]
- connectedness – being connected to others in relationships where you experience joy, can talk and feel understood, and get support[28]
- positivity resonance – the experience of shared feelings and caring for another
- larger social networks – having a sense of belonging and support through access to a greater number of social connections
- physical activity – having a regular exercise routine and regularly spending time outdoors.

The report highlights how these key protective factors have supported people during the pandemic towards positive wellbeing. It also outlines the risk factors that may have contributed to negative wellbeing during the COVID-19 pandemic, including not coping well with uncertainty, pre-existing mental health conditions, loneliness, and financial insecurity. For such individuals it is an important priority to manage these important and immediate needs first.

The research so far is showing that while for some people the pandemic has worsened their wellbeing, there are others that are faring better. These findings are encouraging as they reinforce it may be possible to take actions that can better support us to cope with life's challenges and find more joy right now.

Regular reflection may support your agency, learning and growth. You can reflect by stopping and considering your current experience, noticing what comes up for you, considering learnings or information that may help. I invite you to take a few minutes now and reflect on how the COVID-19 pandemic has impacted you and what actions or practices you found helpful, below or in your workbook:

_____

_____

_____

_____

By becoming aware of what you have found helpful, you are beginning to move forward with some clarity around what you should continue to do to support your wellbeing. This awareness will address feelings of languishing. It will strengthen your hope and action to thrive now. This may involve continuing some of your current practices, doing more of them, and considering some new ones.

By doing this you are not ignoring the bad, the pain or the loss. It is all part of your journey moving forward. There may be times you start to feel fatigued, or feel like your mental health is backsliding. This is a normal and natural response to your current circumstances and how your mental health and wellbeing can change. You can, however, rely on the wellbeing plan you will create, to shift you forward towards inner peace, calm, clarity and happiness.

How Am I Feeling Right Now?

I have been working on and prioritising my wellbeing. I continue to make changes as I assess my energy and mindset. As I write this during yet another lockdown in Melbourne, I have felt my energy sliding back again. It was around 80%, but now I feel it is back around 50% of what is normal for me.

I am mindful of staying the course with my self-care. I have re-prioritised and let go of some tasks and projects. I have introduced more positive practices throughout my day, such as stopping to breathe. I continue to have faith that whilst I am finding today not full of ease, I can still work towards improving this situation.

It has been such a long year for many of us, but it can also be an opportunity for reflection, renewal and growth. I am inspired by the mental imagery of a butterfly emerging from its cocoon. In this time of challenge, uncertainty, and change, perhaps there is an opportunity to transform and to do things differently. There is an opportunity for growth through adversity, to reflect, and to be flexible; to be more aware of the fragility of life and time we have, with the extra motivation to *be* in your life with more joy and purpose.

The COVID-19 pandemic has sharpened my focus on what matters most is – MY wellbeing. If we don't take care of ourselves, how can we lead a life of joy, peace and clarity? How do we then take care of others, connect, show our love and provide support? Prioritising myself has helped me learn to tolerate and adjust to life's changes and uncertainties.

Taking care of yourself is possible during challenging times, and so necessary right now. Even during the ebb and flow of our daily lives and emotions we can move towards practices that renew and support our mental health and wellbeing.

The path to wellbeing is not always linear and smooth. It has certainly not been a smooth journey for me. I have felt the lows, frustrations, fears and loss. I have had days where I just wanted to stay in bed and not face the world. I have cried and I have laughed. Importantly, I have also grown. I have taken actions that I never dreamed were possible, such as writing this book, launching an online school, producing a podcast,[1] and maintaining my

---

[1] The *Wellness Solutions* podcast hosted by Mary Mangos, is available at https://www.coachuwellness.com.au/podcast.

boundaries and discipline with my self-care plan. I have learnt it is possible to experience positive growth during difficult times.

My growth includes feeling calmer and happier; even whilst living in a world full of uncertainty. I have learnt to seek more support, maintain my boundaries and say 'no'. I have become more comfortable with shifting my priorities and timings for projects, because I am my first priority. Make yourself your number one. Being number one is not a selfish act. It is an act of love and it is necessary right now. My hope is that as you continue to explore the chapters ahead, you find a practice that lifts you up, calms you down and brings you joy. You can achieve your goals and thrive. Start now!

Inspiration to Cultivate the State of Your Well-*BEing*

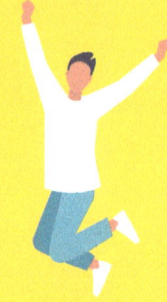

Self-care practices during the COVID-19 pandemic that supported me towards well-*BEing* included:

- more meditation
- more breaks whilst working
- exercising regularly
- better nutrition
- ensuring my news exposure was limited
- staying connected with loved ones
- getting support from medical and mental health professionals
- taking time off work.

You can put the brakes on your stress by normalising how you view uncertainty and increasing your sense of control and agency, to protect and promote your well-*BEing*. Here are some ideas to consider:

- Focus on what you are grateful for by noticing your blessings and expressing appreciation. Try listening to a gratitude meditation.

- Take time to journal and reflect on your resilience and mindset. Identify what community or social resources you can use to get back to coping or thriving.
- Reflect on how well you are doing to just get through your day and week. Our grit has been tested during this time of stress and adversity.
- Look for activities where you in the flow. Get the benefits of feeling immersed, happy and in control of your activities.
- Stay connected with loved ones that support you to feel joy, where you can talk, feel understood, and get the support you need.
- In particular, focus on the interpersonal connections that provide 'positivity resonance'. Shared laugher or smiles, and caring for one another is an important experience that benefits our wellbeing.
- Stay connected to your social networks in your community to maintain a sense of belonging and support.
- Engage in regular physical activity and spend time outdoors to support your physical and psychological wellbeing.

CHAPTER 2
Find Your Energy Zen

*'There is nature and energy in
everything we do and all that we are.'*
Adrienne Posey

Moving slowly, Belinda gets out of bed. She realises that it is Wednesday and there are still three more workdays to go. Quickly running through what she needs to get done today makes her want to curl up back in bed: getting the kids to childcare, remembering to call and check on her mum (who has recently been diagnosed with dementia), and wondering how she will get through all of her work tasks today. 'If I skip lunch and my walk, I may get through some of these priorities,' she thinks. But working through everything feels so hard. So many distractions get in the way, including her worries and thoughts about all the other things she needs to get done.

If you can connect with Belinda's story, then you are among many who feel this way. We have endured more change and uncertainty during the COVID-19 pandemic than many of us have experienced in several years, collectively. It is easy to see why we might be feeling exhausted and distracted, with barely enough energy to make dinner before collapsing into bed at night. Energy is vital and understanding how to manage your energy is important for your wellbeing and your productivity at work and in life. It is vital that you are aware of the signals you receive, such as fatigue and stress. They provide valuable information about how you are tracking.

Is there something you can do about your energy? Yes, absolutely! First, let's increase your awareness of what supports it. There are important dimensions that support our energy and our well-*BEing*, including:

- essential factors like sleep, exercise and diet
- self-care practices like meditation, taking breaks and reflection
- emotions from practices like gratitude, our connections and purpose.

Most of us can extend our energy beyond the 'recommended' when necessary. Pushing ourselves a little more at the gym, getting less sleep due to a sleepless child or illness in the family, an occasional late night, or having an extra bowl of dessert every so often are not likely to significantly deplete our energies on their own. It is when we continually push ourselves and exceed our reserves, expecting our bodies and minds to cope, that it may become unsustainable.

FIND YOUR ENERGY ZEN

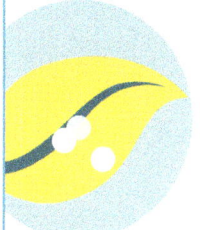

ESSENTIAL FACTORS:
Sleep
Exercise
Diet

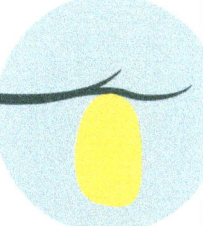

SELF - CARE:
Meditation
Breaks
Reflection

EMOTIONS:
Gratitude
Connections
Purpose

SOURCE: MARY MANGOS @COACHUWELLNESS

Find Your Energy Zen

If you feel your energy can be improved, or you would like to learn how to consistently manage your energy, then get ready to explore your current state, and understand the essential factors, self-care and emotions practices that can support you. Zen teacher Roshi Susan Murphy explains that 'Zen is the practice of agreeing to live with a mind and self as alive and fluid as breathing itself: accepting the offer of each moment, yielding to the passing of each moment.'[29] To support this practice, I am encouraging you to begin first by exploring your energy and prioritising practices that may support you. My reference to 'energy zen' is all about the foundations that support your ability to feel more at ease, become more accepting and find more joy in your current circumstances.

Let's begin by assessing your energy right now. It involves beginning with an energy awareness exercise before exploring how to cultivate your mindful awareness towards a life of ease and peace. Check the statements 'yes' or 'no' as you consider how they apply to you below or in your workbook. The more yes's you have checked on your list, the better the foundations for your well-*BEing*:

ESSENTIAL FACTORS	Yes/No
I go to bed and wake up the same time each day.	
I avoid caffeine after 2pm.	
I get outside in the sun for 15 minutes every morning.	
I work out at least three times per week (cardio).	
I do some form of strength training at least once per week.	

	Yes/No
I pay attention to my body and how it responds to what I eat.	
I focus on eating whole foods and plant-based foods as a daily foundation.	
I limit sugar and alcohol.	

SELF-CARE	Yes/No
I meditate daily to cultivate mindfulness and peace.	
I focus on one task at a time.	
I take short breaks between tasks.	
I walk outside daily, taking some time to connect mindfully with what I notice and feel.	
When I eat my meal, I take the time to notice and appreciate what I am eating.	
When I'm not at work, I can switch off totally from thinking about work.	
I sit in the morning for at least a few minutes to get centred.	
I regularly reflect on my achievements and progress.	

EMOTIONS	Yes/No
I feel that I have so much in life to be grateful for.	
I am grateful for how my life is now because of the efforts of others.	
I take time to reflect on what I am thankful for.	
I have some strong and deep relationships.	
I have important and valuable connections in the community.	
I spend enough time doing what I need and want to do to make me happy.	
I enjoy making a positive difference to others.	
I engage in pursuits that I am passionate about.	

How to Reflect on Your Energy

Once you complete your assessment of your energy, reflect on the following questions below or in your workbook:

What is working well for me?

It is important to identify this and continue to make time for the energy practices that support your well-*BEing*.

What do I need to do more of?

This question helps you to reflect on what is working well but you would benefit from doing it more often or more consistently. For example, perhaps you have occasionally practiced meditation, but only do it ad hoc. Identify what would be your desired outcome. If you have practiced only monthly, perhaps a weekly goal would be a great place to start for improved well-*BEing*.

What would I like to do differently?

Consider what might be missing that could be supportive of your energy, such as more sleep or spending more time outdoors. Create a list of areas you would like to improve and identify as your first priority.

Before you begin to consider how you might work on what is a priority for you, consider the following ideas. As you explore them in each section – essential factors, self-care, and emotions – pause and reflect on what ideas support your priorities.

Essential Factors for Well-*BEing*

- Enhance your sleep by setting an earlier bedtime, reducing your alcohol intake, eating dinner earlier, limiting the use of electronic devices in your bedroom, and some deep breathing as you count.
- Eat nutritious meals and snacks through the day.
- Engage in cardiovascular activity three times per week and strength training once per week for stress release.
- Learn to notice signs of imminent energy flagging, such as restlessness, yawning, hunger, and lack of focus on tasks.

From the above list, what resonates for you?

Self-care for Well-*BEing*

- Take regular, brief breaks away from your desk at 90–120-minute intervals throughout the day.
- Reduce interruptions by performing high-concentration tasks away from emails and phones.
- Try practices like meditation or deep breathing.
- Every night, identify the most important challenge for the next day then make it your priority for when you begin the next morning – but park it until then.

From the above list, what resonates for you?

Emotions for Well-*BEing*

- Defuse your feelings of irritability, impatience, anxiety, and insecurity through slow, deep abdominal breathing.
- Fuel positive emotions within yourself and others by regularly expressing appreciation to others in detailed, specific terms, such as notes, emails, calls, or conversations. Notice the good!
- Look at negative situations through a new lens.
    - Adopt a 'reverse lens' to ask, 'What would the other person in this conflict say and how might they be right?'
    - Use a 'long lens' to ask, 'How will I likely view this situation in six months?'
    - Employ a 'wide lens' to ask, 'How can I grow and learn from this situation?'

From the above list, what resonates for you?

Remember that it is normal to struggle, especially during uncertain and challenging times. Avoid the urge to just manage your time better and get more done in your day. Reflect on your energy in an integrated way that includes the essentials, self-care and emotions. That is the key to finding actions that make a positive difference for you.

Inspiration to Cultivate Your Well-*BEing* by Enhancing Your Energy Zen

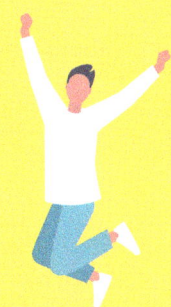

- Take time to explore your current state and understand what impacts your energy.
- Complete the energy awareness exercise.
- Make note of what is depleting your energy and what is filling your tank.
- Consider your essential factors — are you getting enough good-quality sleep? Are you eating fresh, nutritious food? Are you getting enough exercise?
- What self-care actions can you try? Are you taking breaks for yourself?
- Are you connecting to positive emotions like gratitude? Or are you fuelling negative emotions that drain you?

CHAPTER 3
Cultivating mindful Clarity

'Your mind's natural state is one of clarity and luminosity. And so, if you engage in the process of developing it, you will be able to see as you have never seen before.'
His Holiness the Gyalwang Drukpa

Looking again at her alarm clock, Mary notices it's 3.17am. The realisation that she hasn't fallen asleep yet stirs up tension and stress in her stomach. 'Why can't I just stop these worries and thoughts running through my mind?' she wonders. Soon she will have to get up and start her day, feeling less than her best and wondering how she will get it all done.

Can you relate to Mary? I know I can, because Mary was me! As long as I can remember, during the day and often when I tried to sleep at night, I would worry and ruminate about what had happened, what people said, what I should have said, what I needed to do and how I might fail. Eleven years ago, I found my pathway back to steadiness, calm and clarity. This happened for me through mindfulness and meditation practice.

Practicing mindfulness benefits you by strengthening your emotional control, so you can better deal with uncertainty and stress, and all that it brings you on a day-to-day basis. It increases your awareness of your inner critic and finding ease and agency when you become unsettled or confused. There may be times when you feel like another being has inhabited your mind and taken control. Natalie Goldberg, in her book *Writing Down the Bones,* describes her experience of this inner voice, this inner critic, in a very familiar way:

> 'Don't be tossed away by your [inner critic]. You say you want to do something—"I really want to be a writer"—then that little voice comes along, "but I might not make enough money as a writer." "Oh, okay, then I won't write."'[30]

I struggle with this from time to time; I stare at my screen, filling my brain with defeat even before I begin. In particular, this can occur for me when I do something challenging and new. If you become aware of your mind's chatter and overthinking, consider a calming practice that acknowledges and proactively enhances your awareness of how you feel and what you pay attention to. One way you can do this is by cultivating your mindfulness.

What Is Mindfulness?

Mindfulness is an every-day experience where you pay attention to one thing at a time. This could be when you cook your dinner, focusing on the ingredients, how they look and smell. It could be when chatting to a loved one, as you listen to what they are communicating.

> *'Mindfulness is the awareness that arises from paying attention, on purpose, in the present moment, and non-judgmentally.'*
> **Dr Jon Kabat-Zinn**

It is perfectly normal to feel distracted. Research has shown that about half of the time (47%), we are not really paying attention to what's going on around us.[31] Unless you have to focus on a recipe, most of us are likely to chop, sauté, dice, dress a salad, and serve it up without really thinking about it step by step. But one study from Harvard University reported that people are happier when their mind is not wandering from what they are doing.[32]

You might have a task to complete and find that your mind wanders toward another task that needs starting, or towards where you wish you were instead, or to some problem that happened in the past, or back to other thoughts and worries in your life. When you move away from the present, you do not feel happier. Instead, it serves to activate centres in the brain that may cause or prolong your stress response.

From a neuroscience point of view, you may have 'wired in' this pattern of behaviour – which means you can 'unwire' it. The more you notice your thoughts and choose which ones that you focus on, the stronger your circuits get. One way to do this is through meditation.

Why Is Meditation Helpful for Your Well-*BEing*?

Meditation is a way to train the brain and strengthen your mindfulness. Studies suggest that mindfulness meditation can positively impact your psychological and physical wellbeing, and have shown that the brain's grey matter is thicker in areas associated with the senses, memory and executive function in long term mindfulness meditators. One such study used magnetic resonance imaging to assess cortical thickness after an 'insight meditation experience', and found 'that regular practice of meditation is associated with increased thickness in a subset of cortical regions related to somatosensory, auditory, visual and interoceptive processing.'[33]

The initial results of these studies suggest that meditation may be associated with structural changes in areas of the brain that are important for sensory, cognitive and emotional processing. How amazing it is that! Your brain can change in ways that supports you to move away from unhelpful patterns of 'wandering off' and worrying. Instead, through regular practice, you begin to strengthen what you notice, how you feel and how you solve your problems. This means you can tone down or even change the meaning you place on something, lessening your reaction to it, and if it's an arresting or shocking situation, your recovery from it may be more resilient.

With less 'wandering off', more strengthening of what you pay attention to and how you respond, also comes clarity, self-control and improved agency. Having clarity around what is important for you to focus on and why it matters to you, can provide you with reassurance around your purpose. The self-control to work on what is important right now, despite distractions and temptations, is key for many of us to achieve goals that matter. Writing this book would not have been possible without my every-day mindfulness meditation practice which supports me to maintain my self-control and manage other priorities, temptations and distractions.

If you would like to work on cultivating your mindful clarity, let's first begin with some reflection to consider. Reflection is an important part of mindfulness practice through improved awareness of its impact, new benefits and what you wish to change. Consider your responses to each of the following questions, or just select one or two questions that resonate for you. If you need to pause here, remember to take all the time you need. Use the section below or your workbook.

What goals and dreams do I have that I feel are being diverted by being on autopilot?

Do I over-analyse situations? What are some recent examples?

Is it hard for me to stop worrying? What kind of things do I worry about?

Do I feel I am missing a sense of achievement and progress with what is important to me?

How does this impact me?

What changes do I wish to see?

The next step is to cultivate your mindfulness practice. This involves four steps: *setting your intention, embracing uncertainty, welcoming all emotions,* and *moving towards peace and joy.* Have a look at the next image for a visual representation.

CULTIVATING MINDFUL CLARITY

Set Your Intention

Embrace Uncertainty

Welcome All Emotions

Move Towards Peace & Joy

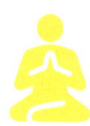

SOURCE: MARY MANGOS @COACHUWELLNESS

Let's Explore How to Cultivate Mindful Clarity

Set Your Intention

Setting an intention is like making a promise to yourself to focus and work towards what you want to happen. When I decided I had enough of the ruminating and worrying, I made a promise to myself that I could be calm, I could have clarity and focus and this would show up with my productivity and progress at work and in my relationships. To identify your intention:

- Consider your **WHAT?** What do you desire to be happening that would indicate that your life or situation is now improved or ideal? For example, feeling calmer and more focused at work.

- Get **SPECIFIC**. Identify specific short-term actions or behaviours that you want to grow. Here is some inspiration: to prioritise yourself more; to have more compassion; to increase your joy; to feel more aligned to what matters to you; to feel more peace; or to find beauty in everything.

- Remember that your intentions can **EVOLVE** and grow. For example, we may start with an intention of growing our own self-compassion. When you feel you are living this intention more comfortably, this may evolve towards compassion for others we care about and those we find challenging.

Write your intention here or in your workbook:

Embrace Uncertainty

We don't live in a bubble. Instead, we are always interacting with people and the world, and this interaction may be impacting our thoughts, feelings and our actions. Not knowing what might happen tomorrow or even today may cause us feelings of fear and frustration. I believe it is possible to feel comfortable and even happy with uncertainty. To accept whatever may unfold and have faith that all will be well is possible. One way you can become more comfortable with uncertainty is by letting things unfold with a flexible mindset. Having a mind that responds flexibly can support your happiness and help you to achieve your intentions.

One strategy to support your flexibility with uncertainty is to cultivate a 'don't know mind' for more openness and contentment amid uncertainty.

A 'don't know mind' works this way:[34]

- Bring to your mind a conflict or a situation you've experienced.
- Allow your awareness to explore all the thoughts, feelings and opinions you have about that conflict or situation, and how it should be.
- Realise that you don't know how the situation should be, will be, or what might happen. Say to yourself: 'I don't know.'
- Consider how having no fixed opinion and complete openness makes you feel.
- As new thoughts, feelings or opinions come up, keep saying: 'I don't know.'
- Keep doing this until you are comfortable with the uncertainty; until you can smile or even laugh when you say 'I don't know.'

By practicing a 'don't know mind', you can begin to see yourself coping better with uncertain or stressful situations. You begin to imagine that something better might be also about to happen. Might it be a good thing to miss out on this job, house, or opportunity, because something better could be lining up for you? Simply imagine from a point of 'I don't know' and see what unfolds for you. You can also listen to my 'don't know mind' meditation at https://www.coachuwellness.com.au/meditations.

Write down your experience of practicing a 'don't know mind' here or in your workbook

Welcome All Emotions

Our emotions are important as they remind us what matters and what actions we should take. For example, if you are considering a new job offer and something doesn't feel right, you might choose to reject the job. Emotions can trigger physical reactions, designed to inform you to further evaluate this situation. They provide useful information that you can reflect on and prioritise. Taking the time to reflect on your emotions is the first step to understanding what you are feeling. This is a mindful experience in itself.

It can sometimes feel challenging to put your feelings into words. Having an emotions wheel can help you to put a name to what you are feeling. Plutchik's Wheel of Emotions identifies eight primary emotions: anger, anticipation, disgust, fear, joy, sadness, surprise and trust. You may identify one of the core words, or the emotions that bookend each core emotion. You will also note the wheel contains emotions that are positioned outside the flower shape too. Have a look at the wheel and explore all the emotions that are possible.

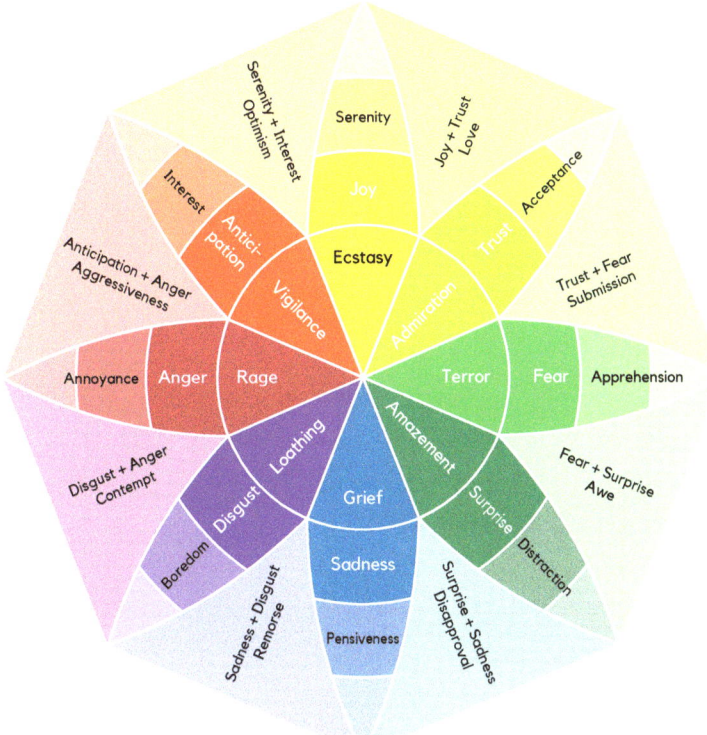

Source: 'The Emotion Wheel: What It Is and How to Use It', PositivePsychology.com[35]

Write down what emotions you are feeling right now.

It may be helpful to become curious and patient with your emotions when you identify and understand your thoughts and feelings. You can cultivate this curiosity and patience, with self-compassion and kindness. When you have compassion and kindness for yourself, you notice your suffering and pain. You realise it is part of the shared experience.

> 'Self-compassion is one of the most powerful sources of strength, coping and resilience we have.'
> **Kristin Neff**

Explore your emotions with this approach (opposite or in your workbook):

Bring to mind a difficult situation and consider what emotions you felt. Use the wheel of emotions to identify one or more emotions that you may have felt.

Then focus on the impact those emotions had on you.

How did that make you act or behave?

For example: Were you having difficulty getting tasks done? Was it making you short-tempered?

Next, show yourself some kindness and self-compassion for your feelings and the experience you are having. Instead of having critical thoughts and wondering why you felt this way, put your hand on your heart and speak to yourself in a way that generates feelings of care.

What can you say to yourself that is kind and compassionate?

Consider some of the following, or create your own below or in your workbook:
- 'It makes sense that I feel worried right now.'
- 'I did the best I could.'
- 'This too shall pass.'

Move Towards Peace and Joy

Creating a mindful life that is full of peace and joy should be a priority. How? You can do this by being aware of how mindful your life is right now. Then, if required, you can work on your ability to cultivate peace and joy, with self-compassion and kindness. Explore if one of the four following options can support your quest for a mindful life.

- **Attending to your life.** Notice the details of your everyday actions. If you're sitting in the passenger seat of a car as someone else drives, you can choose to become mindful in this moment by counting all the red cars you see, or counting a particular make of vehicle. On this journey pay attention to the weather, the traffic, your driver, and how you feel, to increase your mindful awareness. In your interactions with others, look for the beauty in those connections. Really listen and explore what you hear. Try summarising or paraphrasing what you hear. This cultivates your mindfulness, clarity and focus.

- **Take a walk** and pay attention to the sounds that you hear. Don't get caught up with whether you find them pleasant or unpleasant. Shift your awareness to your sense of smell. Again, simply notice. Then move your attention to what you see. Notice each different objects, colour and texture in your environment.

- **Breath counting** can also help to ground you into the present. Slowly inhale, and as you exhale, count 'one' to yourself. Then inhale again and the next time you exhale, count 'two'. Continue to inhale and count on the exhale, until 'five'. You can repeat this as many times as you like until you feel you have more clarity and peace.

- Finally, try **meditation.** There are many amazing meditation apps, YouTube videos, and teachers available if you wish to learn and practice meditation. Given this is one of my favourite practices, I have created several mindful meditations that you can explore.[2] Alternatively, put on some relaxing music on and try the following ...

- Sit in your chair, with an upright but relaxed spine and close your eyes.
- Feel your feet flat on the floor.
- Put your hands on your lap, palms facing upwards.
- Take a deep breath into your stomach, feel your rib cage expand.
- Slowly breathe out.
- Do this again two more times.
- Now allow your breath to settle.
- Follow your breath as it enters your nose or mouth and flows into your body.
- If you find you become distracted with your thoughts, allow them to come and go with kindness. Imagine your thoughts like clouds in the sky floating away.
- Sit following your breath for 5 minutes or more.
- End your meditation by bringing your awareness to your full body, notice how you are feeling, and then open your eyes.

Record your experiences with these practices opposite or in your workbook:

---

[2] These meditations are available at the Coachuwellness website, at https://www.coachuwellness.com.au/meditations.

Attending to your life:

Mindful walking:

Breath counting:

Meditation:

For me, being mindful in my life and meditating daily is essential for my peace and joy. It has become an indispensable part of my physical and psychological wellbeing. Let your intentions lead you on your path to embrace uncertainty, welcome all emotions with kindness and compassion. May it support you towards improved clarity, peace and joy.

Inspiration to Cultivate Mindful Clarity for Well-*BEing*

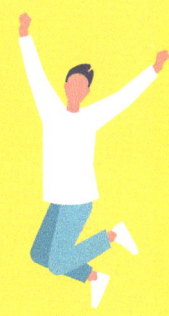

- Strengthen what you pay attention to, to develop more mindful clarity, self-control and improved agency.
- Consider your current state of mindfulness and how your current life practices and thinking impact you.
- Set intention to guide your actions.
- Embrace the uncertainty in your life with a 'don't know mind', to respond flexibly and with ease.
- Welcome all of your emotions by putting your feelings into words using the 'Plutchik's Wheel of Emotions'.
- Cultivate more peace and joy by noticing everyday actions, mindful walking, breath counting and meditation.

CHAPTER 4
Happiness Through Gratitude

'Be content with what you have, rejoice in the way things are. When you realise there is nothing lacking, the whole world belongs to you.'

Lao Tzu

As Vanessa sat in her small apartment working during the COVID-19 pandemic lockdown, she found it hard to keep focused on the tasks at hand. She was worrying about how long lockdown would continue and whether this would be just an ongoing part of life now. She could not imagine life as it once was. 'I think I need to lower the bar of joy and happiness,' she thought, 'so I can get on with my life.' Vanessa found it challenging to see things going well in her life now or into the future. She felt a deficit in her agency. The small space she had to live in and now work in meant that the boundaries between her personal and professional life were blurred. Switching off was now challenging as she lived and worked in the same confined space, and she was feeling constantly unhappy.

Vanessa was not alone in feeling that way. According to the Australian Government's Mental Health Commission, '[t]he COVID-19 pandemic is posing significant health, lifestyle and economic challenges for Australians and evidence shows there is likely to be a significant negative mental health impact as a result.'[36]

These mental health challenges are a global experience, with research demonstrating the impact of the pandemic and lockdowns on mental health and wellbeing (see Chapter 1). Even if we cannot change our circumstances, we can still feel joy and happiness. We can do this by moving our focus on something we can control ... our **gratitude**.

Gratitude is not a new concept. It involves thankfulness and appreciation, and is a core practice in many religions and spiritual practices. I can remember being taught by my mum as a young girl to put my hands in prayer position before going to sleep, and give thanks for what I was grateful for. A grateful attitude is critical: supporting our happiness, providing us with energy, hope and the healing that we need to navigate our life.

Cultivating and focusing on your ability to be grateful is an important step towards having and maintaining the inner strength to persevere through tough times and to have hope for positive outcomes. Especially when it feels like negative emotions are gaining momentum and your thoughts are regularly on loss, uncertainty and your anxiety. Having gratitude does not mean that there is no pain, loss or suffering; it is about recognising that there is good around you. By doing so, this can support your health and wellness.

Positive psychology research has reinforced the positive impact that cultivating gratitude can have on our emotions, happiness and general wellbeing, demonstrating that 'positive emotions, including gratitude, are symbiotic with health and wellness, such that positive emotions promote happiness and flourishing, creating an upward spiral.'[37]

In a summary of the findings of research on gratitude and wellbeing, Professor Robert Emmons, the world's leading scientific expert on gratitude, notes that people who participate in intentional gratitude exercises have been found to:

- exercise more regularly
- experience better-quality sleep
- be more likely to have made progress towards an important goal
- report higher levels of positive moods and states, including enthusiasm, optimism and determination
- have an improved sense of connection with others, and help or offer support to others more often.[38]

When you are feeling grateful, your attention is shifted from your negative emotions. For someone like Vanessa, cultivating more gratitude would make it harder for her to ruminate on her negative feelings about working from home, and may help her cope better with the stress and uncertainty of an ongoing lockdown.

I personally love the way gratitude enhances my mood, energy and motivation. I feel more connected to my purpose when I feel grateful. As someone who can easily lean towards pessimistic thoughts, gratitude supports me to feel optimistic and more connected to the important relationships in my life. Even when those relationships have their ups and downs, I can identify and choose to shift toward positive emotions. This supports me to understand and work on issues or problems from a grateful lens.

To create an upward, positive gratitude spiral that can support your well-*BEing* and help you to thrive, let's start with a gratitude awareness exercise. Begin by reflecting on your own current level of gratitude, so that you have an awareness of what is working well and what you might need to do to bring an attitude of gratitude into your every-day life. And let's just be clear here, positive people living in an attitude of gratitude still have to work at it every day. There are down days and sad times that we all feel. In those moments and days, you are encouraged to honour and respect those emotions. Gratitude can then support you to choose your path forward.

Reflect and write down your thoughts for each of the following statements opposite or in your workbook:

1. What do I have in my life that I am thankful for?

2. When I look at the world, I am grateful for...

3. What have people done in my life that I am grateful for?

4. Imagine you are at the end of your life, and as you look back you feel truly grateful for a life well-lived. What has happened to contribute towards that feeling?

Well done completing your reflections. You are on your way towards a peaceful, thriving and happy life. Take a few moments now to write down your learnings from your reflections:

What have I learnt about myself and my life?

What should I continue to do?

What should I do differently?

How did it feel to even consider these questions?

Remember, you can always come back to these questions as you assess how far you have come and where you might like to go next.

The next step is to cultivate your happiness through gratitude with four key practices.

HAPPINESS THROUGH GRATITUDE

3 GOOD THINGS

At the end of your day, before you go to sleep, write down three good things that went well for you that day.

GRATITUDE LETTER

Write a heartfelt letter of gratitude and read it out to that person.

GRATITUDE WALK

While walking, pay attention and notice the positive sights, sounds or smells. Consider why they are positive for you.

GRATITUDE MEDITATION

Begin your day by taking a few deep breaths and connecting with what you are grateful for. Make this your daily mindfulness practice.

SOURCE: MARY MANGOS @COACHUWELLNESS

Increase Your Happiness and Wellbeing Through Gratitude: Four Key Practices

Let's explore each of these practices.

Practice 1 – 3 Good Things:
Every night for one week before you go to sleep, take five minutes to write down **three** things that went really well in your day. Reflect on how you felt about each of them, and then on why they happened. This will help to reinforce and connect your positive emotions to the good things that have happened.

Here is an example. Imagine a friend dropped off some dinner for you. She knows you haven't had a home-cooked meal in a while and wanted to surprise you. That evening, you might write down as one of your good things:

'My friend Beverly dropped off my favourite meal, cannelloni. I didn't expect it and it made me feel loved and appreciated. It happened because we regularly support each other.'

What you notice and identify as one of your three good things doesn't have to be special or a major accomplishment. There are so many ordinary events and experiences that happen in life that are beautiful and meaningful. Here is some inspiration for you to consider:

- 'I drove home and the traffic was lighter than I expected. It felt peaceful for a change.'
- 'The weather report said it would rain, but the sun is out at the moment. I love how it feels on my face.'

- 'My kids laughed so hard in their bath tonight. It gave me so much joy in that moment.'

To begin your practice, write some ideas in the space below or in your workbook. Then try to continue it nightly for a week with the pages provided in your workbook.

3 GOOD THINGS

SOURCE: MARY MANGOS @COACHUWELLNESS

Practice 2 – Write a Gratitude Letter:
Write a heartfelt letter of gratitude to someone thanking them for something they do or did, or an impact they have had on your

life, now or in the past. The letter can affirm the positive things in your life and will remind you of how other people love and care for you. Arrange a time to meet – either online, by phone or in person – and read the letter to them. While you read it, pay attention to their reaction – and to your own responsive reaction. This is a powerful way to boost your relationships (why stop at only one letter?) but also gets you paying more attention to those around you who inspire your gratitude.

Here is an example of a gratitude letter:

GRATITUDE LETTER

Dear Fiona,

I know that I don't say this nearly as often as I should, but I really wanted to thank you for being such a good friend. If I ever need you, you are there for me and happy to listen when I need to talk. We have both shared the highs and lows of life together, and I never could have got through it all without you!

You are one of the most important people in my life. When I count my blessings, I always think of you. I don't think I could have got through this pandemic without you. When I message you, you always make time to respond and you call me back when you can. Through all the stressors in life, your love and support have been invaluable. I appreciate you more than you know!

Thank you again my wonderful friend. I feel lucky to have you in my life. I love you!

Jayne xxx.

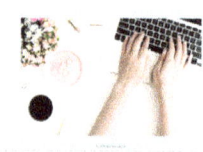

SOURCE: MARY MANGOS @COACHUWELLNESS

Recently, a client of mine let me know what an amazing impact this practice had. She wrote a few letters and called her special people, using Zoom. The first person was so surprised. They didn't expect it and it generated such a nice discussion. The second person she contacted made her feel nervous because they had had some issues in the past. By sharing the letter, she felt such a release and her feelings of gratitude grew and grew. She shared with me:

> '2020 was rough, but it made such a difference counting my blessings with significant others. This meant so much to me and it helped to see so much I am grateful for.'

Gratitude Letter Reflections:
Who would you write to? What will you focus on? When would you do this?

Practice 3 – Take a Gratitude Walk:

How often do you go for a walk and are so immersed in your thoughts that you miss noticing the positive things around you? It is more common than you think. Walking can become a great opportunity to focus on gratitude. This kind of walk is also known as a 'savouring' walk. It involves walking, intentionally noticing the positives around you, and savouring that experience. Research suggests that savouring positive things that we notice, such as trees, flowers and sunshine, can enhance our happiness, boost our gratitude and increases our generosity.[39]

So how can you 'stop and smell the roses'? Try to take a 20-minute walk every day for a week – you can do more or less if that works better for you. During your walk, notice as many positive sights, sounds, or smells as you can. It might include the beauty of the gardens you walk past, or the scent of some flowers nearby, or the sound of children playing happily. Consider why they are positive for you.

A gratitude walk can be done during your normal walk, where you stop along the way. Pausing during your walk regularly creates the opportunities to contemplate and appreciate more in your environment. It provides time to reflect and appreciate what you might see, hear or smell.

Towards the end of your walk, stop and pause again. Take a moment to notice what impact it may have had on you. Do you feel lighter, happier or calmer? Write down some of your thoughts about your walk here or in your workbook.

Gratitude Walk Reflections:

Practice 4 – Do a Gratitude Meditation:
Start your day connecting with gratitude to enhance your wellbeing and increase your awareness of what you are grateful for. Try waking up and making your gratitude practice your first priority. Avoid waking up and reading the news on your phone, scrolling through your social media, or checking your email. Set up your mindset and your wellbeing in the best way possible.

> 'Buddhist monks begin each day with a chant of gratitude for the blessings of their life. Native American elders begin each ceremony with grateful prayers to mother earth and father sky, to the four directions, to the animal, plant, and mineral brothers and sisters who share our earth and support our life.'[40]

Begin by taking a few deep breaths. Breathe in deeply and slowly exhale. Feel any tension melting away. In this relaxed and calm state, reflect on one or two things you are grateful for. It might include your loved ones, the weather today, or the delicious dinner you had last night. As you reflect on what you are grateful for, say 'thank you' for it. Connect with your body and notice where the grateful feelings reside. Take a few breaths and bring that feeling of gratitude with you as you go through your day.

You can also follow a guided meditation as part of your morning practice. If this is something you are interested in, explore my gratitude meditation on my website, at www.coachuwellness.com.au/meditations. Meditation, whether doing your own or listening to a guided practice, can support your agency, help you to stay in the present and focus on actions or feelings that cultivate your gratitude.

After completing your meditation, take a moment to write down what impact it had on you, using your workbook or the section below. This is a great opportunity to understand the value of this practice for you.

Gratitude Meditation Reflections:

This chapter explored four gratitude practices: three good things, gratitude letters, gratitude walks and gratitude meditation. If you are wondering what you should choose as your practice, consider which one of the four resonated most strongly for you. Trust your intuition. Begin with the one that interests you the most and then perhaps try the others later. May your reflections and gratitude practices build your agency, support you to notice the good around you, and build your happiness and wellbeing.

Gratitude Inspiration to Cultivate Your Well-*BEing*

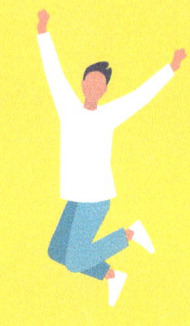

- Focus on your ability to be grateful, to support you to persevere through tough times and have hope for positive outcomes.
- Reflect on what you are thankful for and what has happened to contribute to this feeling.
- Explore four key practices that can make a difference to your well-*BEing*: journal three good things that happened in your day; write a gratitude letter expressing your gratitude to someone; go for a gratitude walk where you notice positive sights, sounds and smells; and do a gratitude meditation.

CHAPTER 5
The Power of Affirmations and Positive Self-Talk

'Optimism is the faith that leads to achievement. Nothing can be done without hope and confidence.'
Helen Keller

How you talk to yourself matters a lot. Have you ever accidentally bumped into something, stubbed your toe, hit your funny bone, and you berated yourself for 'being so dumb' or called yourself a name like 'stupid'? We all do it. It's often feels like a natural reflex to an unexpected action or accident.

What about when you let yourself down with something more serious, like your child falling ill or having an accident? What is the impact on us? I remember so clearly an awful event that happened when my eldest son was two and half years of age and my youngest son nine months old. It had been a difficult transition for me as a mother, going from one child to two. The adjustment was not easy as I was experiencing significant sleep deprivation and getting very little rest during the day.

My husband suggested that we take a short break away from home for a few days to try to renew our energy, leaving our children with my mum. I reluctantly agreed to this idea, and spent the whole time away thinking about how they should be with me and that I was a bad mother for prioritising my own needs over theirs. I brought these feelings of shame back home.

The day after we returned from our short break, my eldest son fell down at home and broke his femur. It was an accident, but I 'beat myself up' over it. I was still carrying the shame of prioritising myself. The shame of not being the perfect mum. I wondered if I could have done something to prevent this horrible accident. All of these thoughts I kept to myself. It affected my emotions and behaviour. I started to do even less for myself as I wanted to prioritise my children even more. This became a dark period for me as I fell into depression. I wasn't ready to embrace seeing myself from a loving lens. I was still punishing myself.

After much reflection and support, I understand that I have made and will continue to make mistakes. I can learn from these and accept my strengths and imperfections. I give myself permission to be human. Giving yourself permission is important as it changes how you see yourself, and the behaviours and actions that support a happier life. Most of us want to see ourselves as competent, compassionate, and worthy.

Do you beat yourself up for being human? Maybe you've developed a belief about yourself that 'you're always late'. Or that 'you are not good enough'. These are a few examples of hundreds of ways we talk ourselves into or out of beliefs about our abilities, behaviours, or even our good fortune.

Negative self-talk and unhelpful behaviours can be challenging to change. This is where affirmations can help. Affirmations (also called 'self-affirmations') are statements said with confidence about a perceived truth. They help people to make significant changes in their lives. An affirmation can work as it can direct your mind into giving more attention towards the stated concept.

In Dr Shauna Shapiro's latest book *Good Morning, I Love You*, she describes how research has shown that we can change our ingrained habits through the power of neuroplasticity. Neuroplasticity refers to the capacity of neurons and neural networks in the brain to change their connections and behaviour in response to new information. When we direct our attention toward positive information, with kindness, compassion and love, we are rewiring our brain. Dr Shapiro explains that '[h]aving the right attitude and intention is essential. Kindness and curiosity serve as basic building blocks for meaningful and lasting change.'[41]

When we are kind and curious with our attitude, we release a cascade of chemicals that turn on the learning centres of our brain. In every moment of our lives, we are practicing and growing something. Being intentional about what we wish to grow allows us to rewire our brain to become happier. When we use affirmations mindfully and with kindness, we are growing something positive. The regions in the brain that are activated in this process are often referred to as the 'reward circuits', and include the medial prefrontal cortex and posterior cingulate cortex.[42] These regions support our planning, decision making, problem solving, self-control, and regulate the balance of internal and externally focused attention. Affirming statements can help our brain to 'wire in' the positive affirmation, and doing this may prime our mindset for positive actions and behaviours.

What Are Affirmations?

Affirmations are positive statements used to increase your positive thoughts and to set an intention for your day. They help to change your internal narrative and unhelpful self-talk. They can positively impact how you feel and the actions you choose to take.

Research into the use and impact of affirmations have found a wide range of positive impacts. Affirmations have been found to:

- decrease health-deteriorating stress[43]
- be used effectively in interventions that led people to increase their physical activity[44]
- make people less likely to dismiss harmful health messages, responding instead with the intention to change for the better[45] and to eat more fruit and vegetables[46]
- lower stress and rumination.[47]

Affirmations can broaden our perspective of ourselves and the situations we might experience. In particular, my interest is in how affirmations can grow our optimism and alter our mindset towards improved clarity about the change you desire. Growing your optimism is valuable, as it can help to support a hopeful outlook about your future. It is more than just feeling good.

> *'Optimism is ... about being engaged with a meaningful life, developing resilience, and feeling in control. This dovetails nicely with psychological research showing that the benefits of optimism come from the ability to accept the good along with the bad, and being prepared to work creatively and persistently to get what you want out of life. Optimistic realists, whom I consider to be the true optimists, don't believe that good things will come if they simply think happy thoughts. Instead, they believe at a very deep level that they have some control over their own destinies.'*
>
> **Professor Elaine Fox**[48]

Optimism doesn't mean ignoring the current situation. As you go about your day, you experience the joys, changes, surprises and challenges. As you navigate your experience, you can accept our current circumstances and still feel hopeful and confident about the future. It is possible to be grounded in your experience right now, have compassion for yourself and also move towards your hopes and dreams. If you are ready to foster your optimism, let's explore my process of creating affirmations.

My process is inspired by cognitive behavioural therapy (CBT) in the way I like to create and use my affirmations. The key focus of CBT is that thoughts, feelings and behaviours combine to influence a person's quality of life. The CBT model '"hypothesises that people's emotions and behaviours are influenced by their perceptions of events. It is not a situation in and of itself that determines what people feel but rather the way in which they construe a situation" ... In other words, how people feel is determined by the way in which they interpret situations'[49]. CBT focuses on identifying unhelpful thoughts and beliefs, challenging and reframing them, and supporting improved outcomes and behaviours.

Part of my affirmation process encourages you to identify the thoughts, emotions and beliefs that you are troubled with or find unhelpful right now. In addition to increasing your awareness, I will show you how to identify areas to focus on that can support the positive change you desire. Some examples of your thinking that may trouble you:

- 'I don't think my colleagues respect my capabilities at work.'
- 'I will never get fit and feel energetic.'
- 'I am not lucky like others are.'
- 'Nothing good ever happens to me.'
- 'I am getting so old; I can't do anything anymore.'

By identifying YOUR unhelpful thinking, you begin to focus on what you want to change and create the inspiration you will use for what affirmations will best support YOU.

Here is how it works. In the following image, I outline my affirmation steps. They include:

- identifying your priorities to help you to focus on what you want to change
- creating present tense, positive affirmations
- how to use them
- connecting to yourself mindfully.

AFFIRMATIONS FOR YOUR BEST SELF

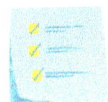

IDENTIFY YOUR PRIORITIES

Start by identifying what is not working well for you. What feelings, thinking or behaviour do you want to change?

CREATE POSITIVE AFFIRMATIONS

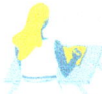

Be affirmative to your negative feelings, thoughts or behaviours to address them positively. Keep them in the present tense, as if they have already happened. "I am calm and confident".

SAY IT OUT LOUD

First thing in the morning read out your affirmation for 5 minutes. Look at yourself in the mirror as you repeat your positive affirmation.

CONNECT TO YOURSELF

Place your hand over your heart as you repeat your affirmation. Take a few deep breaths and notice how your body feels.

SOURCE: MARY MANGOS @COACHUWELLNESS

The First Step Towards Becoming Your Best Self That Prioritises Well-*BEing* ...

- Identify your priorities to help to you to focus on WHAT is not working well and what you wish was better or different. What feelings, thinking or behaviours do you want to change?
- Make a list of what you would like to change and why you wish to change it. Describe the impact it is having on your well-*BEing*, including your thinking, feeling and behaviours. For example:
  'I think that I am not smart enough and it makes me feel like I'm not good enough. I always overthink my proposals at work, I spend far too much time working on them and never feel satisfied.'
- Write them down using the workbook or in the space below. Don't judge yourself by considering if they are true or not. This is an important step as it is the foundation for your affirmative statements.

My priorities — What are they and what do I wish was different?

The Second Step ...

- Focus on one priority and one affirmation at a time.
- Create your affirmation, ensuring it is positive and written in the present tense.
- Using the previous example:
  'I think that I am not smart enough and it makes me feel like I'm not good enough. I always overthink my proposals at work, I spend far too much time working on them and never feel satisfied.'
- Create an affirmation that helps to reverse this:
  'I am smart, I am confident. I complete my work with ease and appreciate my efforts at work.'

Let's Look at Some More Examples of Affirmations:

- 'My relationships are mutually loving and respectful.'
- 'I am grounded, I am peaceful and calm.'
- 'I trust in my ability to be helpful and to be helped when I need it.'
- 'I surrender my need for control.'
- 'My abundance of love flows freely, I am blessed in the giving and receiving of love.'
- 'My skills are highly valuable and sought after by high value companies.'
- 'My lovely new boss is eagerly seeking my special talents now.'
- 'My dream job is now ready for me.'

Remember, the above examples may be helpful to you if they address what YOU are feeling or thinking. If you choose to create affirmations that are broad in their priorities, that's okay too; it may still support you and how you feel. With my exercise, you are connecting with the unhelpful thinking or expectations that you want to shift. By then practicing your new helpful thoughts, the goal is to grow these and support the positive change you are searching for.

How do you know if your affirmations are effective? Go back to your priorities or your reasons for creating them and say your affirmation out loud. Next, pause and reflect. Consider how you feel after you say them. How do they impact your mood or feelings? Even feeling a little more hopeful is a great direction.

Try to scale how you are feeling. You can do this by using a scaling measure of 1 to 10 about your affirmation. For example, with the 'smart and confident' affirmation, 1 would be the lowest possible score and 10 would be the maximum for feeling smart and confident. Rate how you feel prior to and after saying the affirmation. Let's say that prior to the affirmation, you gave yourself a rating of 3 out of 10. What rating would you now give yourself out of 10? When I work with clients, any movement forward along the scale is progress. Even a 5 or 6 initially is a wonderful positive achievement.

Now it's your turn to create an affirmation. Use the workbook or write your response below.

MY AFFIRMATION:

The Third Step ...

Here are some instructions on HOW to use the affirmations you have created.

- In the morning, stand in front of your mirror, repeating the affirmation over and over for 5 minutes.
- Read your affirmation throughout the day. I like to put my affirmation on my phone as a screensaver so that I can look at it regularly throughout my day.
- Keep doing this every day for at least a month, or until you feel it has had a positive impact on your priorities.
- Use the earlier idea of scaling to assess your progress.

The Fourth and Final Step ...

This step supports the third step; how to make the most of your affirmation practice.

- Put your hand on your heart, take a few deep breaths and notice how your body feels while you say your affirmation out loud.
- Connect to yourself mindfully, with love and kindness, as you repeat your affirmation.
- Take a few moments to reflect on your positive journey.
- WELL DONE! You have taken the time to make a difference for yourself.

Because I 'practice what I preach', I love to create affirmations regularly to address how I might be feeling and thinking, and to rewire my brain. I use the one below anytime I am feeling unsafe and fearful about what may be happening in my life, and it was incredibly helpful for me during the COVID pandemic:

> **AFFIRMATION**
>
> I am calm
> I focus on
> what I can
> control
> I let go of
> what I can't
>
> SOURCE: MARY MANGOS @COACHUWELLNESS

I created this second affirmation to respond directly to my negative rumination at the time. I wanted to deal with my own negative self-talk that involved questioning my own capability to support my clients.

> **AFFIRMATION**
>
> I am present
> I have clarity
> I am wise
> I find solutions
> with ease
>
> SOURCE: MARY MANGOS @COACHUWELLNESS

During the first few months of the pandemic, I was driven with the purpose to make a positive difference to others. To improve their mental health, happiness and wellbeing. I had set myself up with high expectations of what I wanted to achieve at work and this produced a negative impact, making me feel unhappy and stressed. I created the following affirmation to encourage a more kind and compassionate response to myself. I also wanted to focus and prioritise my own happiness and health more:

> **AFFIRMATION**
>
> I am being kinder to myself and working towards being the happiest, healthiest version of me.
>
> SOURCE: MARY MANGOS @COACHUWELLNESS

When I say in the above affirmation, 'I am being kinder to myself …', you may wonder why I choose this over, 'I am kind …'. Either phrasing can be effective here, but I consider myself a realistic optimist. I like my affirmations to feel both achievable and hopeful at times, even if I know it might be a process. They work for me as they provide me with something to work towards.

When You Are Finding It HARD!

Remember that a daily affirmation practice has the potential to make a positive difference. If you feel they are not working for you, it could be because new things can be challenging. Perhaps you need to take a step back and acknowledge your current challenges and feelings. Try the following steps:

- When you identify your negative thinking in the first step, take some time to acknowledge how you think and feel. Acknowledge how it impacts you.
- Lean into your kindness and curiosity and ask yourself some questions such as, 'When have I felt good here? When does this not happen for me?' Bring your attention to your reflections so that you shift your mindset into a more creative space for creating affirmations.
- When saying your affirmation out aloud,
  - ask yourself, does it feel hopeful and achievable?
  - repeat it with conviction.
  - imagine that it is already true, and think about how this makes you feel.

- Focus on one affirmation that you value for longer. Take your time working on one area before creating another.
- Show yourself some self-compassion and patience.
- Finally, consider seeing a coach or therapist who can offer you further guidance.

Here is some final inspiration for your affirmations:

- 'I let go and feel at peace.'
- 'My body feels refreshed and my mind is clear.'
- 'I am focused and productive.'
- 'I feel flexible and resilient.'
- 'I prioritise myself with kindness and compassion.'
- 'My heart is filled with joy and peace.'

For more examples of affirmations, please explore my Instagram @coachuwellness.

The use of positive affirmations can change your life, like they have mine. They can reduce your stress and enhance your wellbeing. Create some affirmations today that improve your agency, support you toward positive change and achieve your priorities. Try them now! I hope they help you create the life you desire.

Inspiring Affirmations for Well-*BEing*

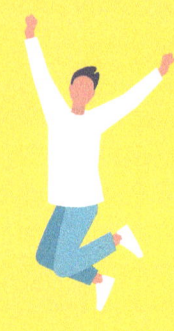

- Positive affirmations can improve your agency, support your priorities and well-*BEing*.
- Affirmations are positive statements that increase positive thoughts and well-*BEing*.
- When you direct your attention towards positive information, with compassion and kindness, you are rewiring your brain.
- When you use affirmations mindfully, you are growing your optimism and mindful clarity.
- Make a list of what you want to change and what you wish was different.
- Create a positive, present tense affirmation that responds to the change you desire.
- Say your affirmations out loud every day.
- Connect to your mind and body as you say your affirmations.
- Lean into self-kindness and curiosity when you are finding it hard.

CHAPTER 6
Spirituality for Wisdom and Peace

> 'We are not human beings having a spiritual experience. We are spiritual beings having a human experience.'
> **Pierre Teilhard de Chardin**

During my youth, I had explored spirituality and prayer for wisdom through my Christian faith. I used my faith and prayer to give thanks, seek guidance to fix my problems and to help me to achieve my goals of doing well at school and in my personal life. But through my 20s, my view of life became much more focused on pleasure. I was creating a life where I tried to maximise the pleasurable aspects of my experiences, which included socialising a lot with friends, eating out, shopping, and travelling when the budget allowed for it.

As I grew and began to earn my own money from part-time jobs, then with full-time professional roles, my desire for 'stuff' began. This extended to what car I drove and my belongings at home. I wanted new and beautiful things for me and for my family. At that time, it was important for me, as someone who came from humble beginnings, to have nice clothes. Growing up with hand-me-downs often left me feeling 'less than' everyone else. I developed a desire to have new things. The state of pleasure I experienced when I bought things helped me to reduce the stress I was feeling at the time, which I was not acknowledging. The joy and peace came for short periods. It did not endure.

It wasn't until after my recovery from depression at age 33 that I started to do more soul searching. I found myself in a far more reflective space, and started questioning my lifestyle, who I was, and what I really wanted from life. *How* did I want to be? How could I take what was good in my life and tap into that to carry me forward? I also reflected on my purpose. It became clear to me that I needed to take a stronger spiritual path that would connect me with the wisdom I needed. I was already connected to my faith and I wanted to further explore what was good for me, what good I needed to do and how to apply it in my life.

As a student at school and university, my attention was always raised when my teachers shared metaphors. Metaphors are amazing as they support comparisons between two unlike things. For example, 'laughter is the best medicine' or 'Sue is an early bird'. One of my favourite metaphors is from Marcel Proust, who wrote, 'Let us be grateful to people who make us happy, they are the charming gardeners who make our souls blossom.' Over the years, metaphors have helped me to understand and visualise unfamiliar concepts. I found them inspiring in their power and influence over my perceptions and emotions. This is why I use them regularly now in my writing and communication to add variety and inspire others' understanding.

I imagine my spiritual wisdom to be a **lotus flower.** This is an image that is so inspiring and beautiful to me that I connect with it regularly. The lotus flower is regarded in many cultures as a symbol of purity, enlightenment, self-regeneration and rebirth. It is the perfect analogy for the human condition – even when its roots are in the dirtiest of waters, the lotus produces the most beautiful flower. That is why I chose it as my business logo, and use it for my website and all of my social media.

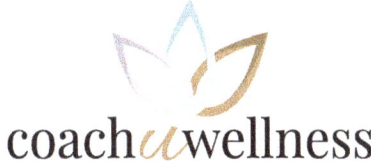

Here is another favourite metaphor that I created and regularly connect with when I pause throughout my day or during meditation to cultivate calm and peace: *'Imagine your worries are clouds passing gently in the sky.'* Like me, I am sure many of you also desire inner peace. This can be triggered from something deeply personal, as it was for me when I was recovering from mental health issues. It can also come from our direct response to our environment. Perhaps the COVID-19 pandemic is taking its toll on you; perhaps you or a loved one has lost their job; perhaps your child is struggling to find their joy.

Organised religion used to be the primary method of seeking solace and calm when life threw us curve balls. Over the past century, it's become more popular and acceptable to borrow concepts from other forms of spirituality to complement and strengthen faith. I see spirituality as an inward journey that may not follow any external rules, one that allows us to adopt a flexible mindset to changes, practices and new ideas.

For me, it is not a choice of one over the other. I believe that both can live in harmony. With or without organised religion, spirituality can support the path towards peace. No matter what your circumstance of challenge, uncertainty or change, you can tap into spiritual wisdom and bloom.

How has it helped me?

- It has helped me to find the peace and comfort that I crave.
- It encourages and reminds me to notice the purpose and meaning in my life.
- It has motivated me to let go, trust in what is here right now and be comfortable with the uncertainty of what may be tomorrow.

Let's explore how others define spirituality and what you can do to begin your spirituality journey.

What Is Spirituality?

'Spirituality has been defined consistently by scientists as the search for or connection with "the sacred". The sacred might be that which is blessed, holy, revered, or particularly special. This can be secular or non-secular: sacredness might be pursued as the search for a purpose in life or as a close relationship with something greater; the sacred might be experienced in the forgiveness offered by a child, a humble moment between a leader and a subordinate, an awe-inspiring sunset, a profound experience during meditation or a religious service, or the self-sacrificing kindness of a stranger.'[50]

I love this definition because it opens up the spirituality realm for all of us. Being in the moment and savouring the amazing and everyday experiences is possible for us all. My favourite everyday experience is watching a beautiful sunset and feeling the peace, joy and awe of being in the moment. What is yours?

Spirituality is also a character strength. Our character strengths are within each of us. When we consider spirituality, we see how it involves the belief that there is a dimension to life that is beyond human understanding. Some of the research on character strengths has included a multi-year research project with the goal of identifying what is best about human beings and how we use these strengths to build the best lives for ourselves and others. This project found that curiosity, zest, hope, gratitude, and **spirituality** were the five key strengths associated with work satisfaction.[51] Another recent study looking at the relationship between spirituality and life satisfaction in Peruvian citizens during the COVID-19 pandemic found that those who had higher levels of spirituality also demonstrated greater life satisfaction.[52]

This research reinforces the importance of spirituality as a driver to your satisfaction. Dr Ryan Niemiec, a leading character-strengths researcher and the Education Director of the VIA Institute on Character, believes that:

> 'spirituality provides a sense of being grounded, increases optimism, and helps provide a sense of purpose for life. All of these benefits also contribute to an overall greater sense of wellbeing.'[53]

If you are craving some support to begin or to continue your path towards spiritual wisdom, take a moment and reflect on your life journey right now to refocus your mind and spirit. It will help you learn more about what you value and what matters to you. Use the workbook or write your responses below.

REFLECTION QUESTIONS TO ASK YOURSELF RIGHT NOW:

How am I living true to myself?

What worries me most about the future?

What do I need to let go of?

What matters most in my life?

What do I want most in life?

When do I feel happiest?

When do I feel at peace?

You can put your spirituality to work by connecting with it as you go about everyday actions in your life. When at work or home, you can reflect on your responsibilities, tasks and conversations. You can connect to the meaning in those sacred moments. This connection to meaning and spirituality can be developed by cultivating a peaceful, calm state. This supports your attention, your awareness and your reflection.

There are two practices that support me to cultivate spirituality – mindfulness and journaling.

SPIRITUALITY FOR WISDOM AND PEACE

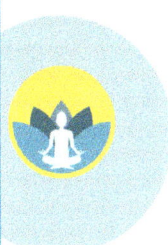

MINDFULNESS:

Practice mindfulness to cultivate calm, peace and clarity

- listen to a guided meditation daily
- set a positive intention
- take a break
- get grounded

JOURNALING:

Start a daily or weekly journaling practice

- reflect on your activities
- record your emotions and feelings
- assess your energy
- reflect on your insights

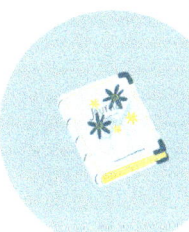

SOURCE: MARY MANGOS @COACHUWELLNESS

Practice 1: Mindfulness

Practice mindfulness to be in the now with your well-*BEing*; to become present with what is important to you. For me, mindfulness is more than just a practice. Mindfulness is a way of life. It's a way of living, noticing, appreciating, staying centred and being well. It keeps me connected to living my life well *now*, and to something greater than myself.

This way of being involves being present and having inner calm on your spiritual journey. Engaging in a daily practice of meditation can help you towards this, and mindfulness meditation in particular can help you to become more aware of yourself.

If you've never tried meditation before, or you aren't sure where to start, there are endless meditation apps available online; my favourite meditation app is the Insight Timer app.[3] Otherwise, there are guided meditations available on my website for you to try.[4] Explore different types of guided meditation to find out what works best for you and what you enjoy.

Here are some tips to help you practice mindfulness and meditation.

- Try to meditate in the morning to begin your day feeling centred and mindful. Alternatively, find another time and place that you can commit to on a daily basis.

---

[3] Information about this app can be found on the Insight Timer website, at https://insighttimer.com.

[4] These meditations can be found on the Coachuwellness website, at https://www.coachuwellness.com.au/meditations.

- Sit or lay down. Do what is most comfortable for you. Because I have chronic issues with my lower back, I enjoy meditating in the morning in bed.
- Don't judge yourself. If you only complete a minute that is okay. If you find your mind and thoughts irritating, just let them come and go. Imagine they are clouds in the sky, floating away.
- After meditation, reflect on how you feel. Is your mind clearer, calmer and more at peace than when you started?
- Identify one or two things that you will do in your day and apply your mindfulness practice to those.
- At the end of your meditation set an intention for your day. For example, your intention might be to notice the positive things that happen to you, or to be kind and more grateful to the special people in your life, or even to see your challenges as opportunities to grow. You can also combine your meditation with intention setting. The gratitude meditation I have on my website is an excellent example of how to meditate and set a positive, grateful intention to your day.
- Plan to have many short, purposeful pauses in your day and they will have a profound impact on your energy, sense of calm, peace and clarity. Try just noticing your breath when you turn your laptop on, or after you check your emails. Do it for a minute and notice how you feel after taking a few breaths in and out mindfully.
- Spend some time in nature every day to increase your calm and reduce your stress. In fact, research has shown

that two hours, spread across the entire week, is an ideal amount of time to be outside. Nature is not only nice to be in, but it is also a must for our health and cognitive functioning.[54] If your desire is to feel calmer, healthier and happier then get out and spend time in parks, forests or fields.

Use the guide below to record your research, your practice, your actions, how you feel, your intentions and behaviours.

MINDFULNESS

Which guided meditations work best for me?

When will I meditate?

How do I feel after I meditate?

What is my intention for the day?

What breaks did I take?

What did I do to get grounded this week?

Practice 2: Journaling

The practice of journaling your reflections about your experiences and what feelings and emotions you had, can help develop your awareness of what you find most engaging and what you find draining. By documenting the present, you rediscover moments that matter to you. Here are my suggestions for how to begin journaling and make it work for you:

- Choose a day and time to reflect. Choose a time during the week that you can have 15-30 minutes of quiet time on a regular weekly basis.
- Think about the activities you were engaged in over the last week, and write down what emotions and feelings you had; e.g., 'I felt a sense of accomplishment getting the report to my supervisor today, even with my kids doing home schooling.'
- Write down how long those emotions lasted.
- Record the energy you feel you gained from your activities as high, medium or low – this will give you a clearer picture of what is draining you and what energises you.
- What have you learnt about yourself?

Use the workbook or the guide opposite to capture your responses to the questions.

JOURNALING

What day and time works best for me?

What emotions and feeling came up for me with the activities I engaged in over the last day or week?

How long did those emotions last?

What was my energy from those activities — was it high, medium or low?

What have I learnt about myself?

I remember when my children were young, it was hard to even think clearly with the busy-ness of life and work. When I journaled and reflected on what brought me joy or energised me, it reminded me of powerful moments of connection with my children. Stopping my focus on tidying up and just playing with my children is what energised me. Building a castle with blocks, reading a book or pushing them on a swing outside; this is what brought me joy. These were my sacred moments that I needed to become more aware of and appreciate in the moment. Journaling and reflection were key to cultivating and sustaining my awareness of what really mattered to me, and has provided me with clarity about my spiritual lessons and priorities. It can for you too!

I see myself as a spiritual student, who keeps an open mind and believes my wisdom will evolve and grow. How has it evolved over the years? Here is **what I have learnt so far on my spiritual journey ...**

- My faith and spiritual practices support my positivity and hope. They support me when my day or week is full of problems or adversities. I can embrace all of my feelings, take the time I need to process them, and have faith that I will be okay. I can get back to feelings of calm and peace.
- I remind myself to prioritise my spiritual journey and reflect regularly on how aligned my decisions and thoughts are with what is important to me. Being aligned involves setting boundaries and reminding

myself regularly of the practices that support me. This is how I stay connected to my journey and have awareness of the sacred moments in my life.
- I like to be spiritually inspired, so I surround myself with the wisdom to grow and learn. I love to do this through prayer, reading books, completing courses, watching webinars from spiritual leaders. My personal favourites include His Holiness the Dalai Lama, Gabrielle Bernstein and His Holiness the Gyalwang Drukpa.
- It is important to be generous and kind with my thoughts, what I communicate and what actions I take. I have learnt to be aware of judgement and the need for control. This has helped me to be aware of giving my love and support to those who might need me in my family, friendship circle, work and our community.
- Finally, sharing my wisdom with others is an important priority that has given me so much joy and happiness. I do this through my writing, my workshops and coaching by listening and supporting others to see what is in their own heart.

I hope my spiritual path inspires you start a journey towards wisdom and peace. May it reduce your stress, and increase your calm and peace. Why not begin now, as your wisdom and peace are already within you. Just look into your heart and be guided.

Spiritual Inspiration for Well-*BEing*

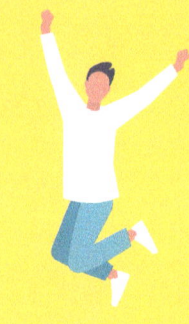

- Reflect on your spiritual path through what matters most to you and when you feel happiness and peace.
- Practice mindfulness to be in the now with your well-*BEing*.
- Listen to a guided meditation daily.
- Identify daily routines that you can do mindfully.
- Take regular pauses in your day and try a breathing exercise.
- Spend time in nature every day for grounding and improved well-*BEing*.
- Practice mindfulness to cultivate calm, peace and clarity.
- Journal regularly to track what energises you and what drains you.
- Consider practices that inspire you, and support your positivity and hope.
- Know that your spiritual wisdom and peace is already within you, ready to guide you.

CHAPTER 7
Your Self-Care Plan

> 'Nourishing yourself in a way that helps you blossom in the direction you want to go is attainable, and you are worth the effort.'
>
> **Deborah Day**

John was not feeling well. He needed to visit his doctor, but he felt he didn't have time. He often felt frustrated at home because he couldn't spend enough time with his family. Often, he felt he couldn't take any holidays with them, because there was too much to do. At work his priority was not failing his customers, resolving any negative feedback and ensuring customer actions were implemented. Keeping others happy was his mission. John was putting himself last! Can you relate to John? I know many of you will. Throughout our time working together, I coached John, and we developed a self-care plan. This plan and the actions to support it helped John to achieve his intentions for a happier, healthier and connected life that was aligned with what mattered to him. John **put himself first** and focused on how to thrive in life and at work. John transformed how he lived his life at home and at work, his wellbeing and his happiness. If you want to do this too ... read on.

In the previous chapters, I have shared strategies that can help you to **blossom in the direction of your well-BEing.** It included focusing on your energy, mindfulness, gratitude, affirmations and spirituality. We are now going to bring it all together with some frameworks to help you create your own self-care plan. And by doing so it will provide the agency you require. Let's begin by defining what it is and why it is important.

'Self-care' means the deliberate actions or activities a person undertakes specifically in order to maintain or increase their wellness and/or their wellbeing.[55] The perspective I take towards **self-care** focuses on how you can look after your own well-*BEing* both professionally and personally. I believe self-care to be a critical priority, because it supports me to maintain my hope and positivity. It also enables me to then support and care for my family, my friends, my colleagues and clients. And now with the impact of the COVID-19 pandemic, we are exposed to more stress. Increased uncertainty, change, heavy workloads, limited support, high demands and ever-increasing expectations in work and life, mean that self-care is vital.

While the concept of 'self-care' has been around for many years, especially in medical and physical health and wellness fields,[56] it has become something of a 'buzzword' recently; either seen as a 'superficial fad', or a term used so broadly that doesn't mean much at all.[57] It is great if you do something like have a bath at night as part of your self-care, but having a broader vision for *how* and *why* that action benefits you can guide you towards the practices that will really make a positive difference to your well-*BEing*. I believe that it isn't enough to just focus on self-care as a practice; it involves conscious, active engagement in *BEing* caring toward yourself.[58]

My vision of a self-care plan rests on four key foundational principles.[59] First, self-care activities should be ones that can be integrated into your life, rather than feeling like an additional burden or stress. Second, self-care activities should be those that build up your wellbeing enough for you to have the capacity to give back to and support others. Third, a self-care plan should be one that is intentionally chosen, engaged with and developed over time, especially as your needs or circumstances change. Finally, and most importantly, a self-care plan should encourage you to take actions that enable you to flourish, not just cope or survive. Surviving means that you are just getting by in life, while focusing on how to reduce or prevent negatives; but when you're flourishing, you become open to possibilities and opportunities, and seek out positive growth and development. This helps you to build a life of meaning and purpose. For me, it also gives me hope that life can be more than just okay. Life can be great, even now. With that in mind, you can prioritise activities that enhance how you feel, and build your resilience and positivity.

How do you do this? By being **intentional** about what you are trying to achieve with your self-care plan. It is not simply a list of things to do. It is your WHY. It explains why you value self-care, what you hope to achieve. For me, my vision is to create a zen life where I feel clarity, peace and calm. This is because I know I have a tendency to become worried and anxious a lot and this impacts my life. It impacts me by limiting my joy and draining my energy. Creating a zen life for me is what will make me happy. It helps me to engage in my life with joy and positivity. It supports me to make a positive difference with my family, friends, clients and the world. So it is crucial that my self-care plan includes those activities and actions that directly lead to and support this vision, and that I leave out activities and actions that don't – even if they feel quite nice in general.

Remember the words from Aristotle:

'The soul never thinks without a picture.'

What is your picture? What is your WHY? It may feel uncomfortable to answer this because it may not be something you have done before. Often, we feel it has to be perfect. Remember, it doesn't. Prepare your mindset for some writing. Do a meditation or go for a walk before starting. Play some calming music. Tell yourself you are just capturing what is important. Define your vision using your workbook or below. Take your time and come back to the questions as often as you need to.

What do I hope my self-care plan will achieve for me? What do I hope to become?

For example: 'I want to create a life where I feel nurtured, secure, safe and loved.' Consider instances in the past where you felt your vision occurred. What actions were you taking at this time?

What areas of my wellbeing would I like to see flourishing?

Here are some ideas:
- boundaries between work and my personal life
- how I respond to stress and adversity
- my physical wellbeing
- being more flexible as my needs change.

The next step is to put it all together and start writing your self-care vision. Consider starting your vision statement with 'I feel [areas of focus] each day' if you need a prompt.

Here are some examples:

- I feel calm and joy every day and I inspire others.
- I prioritise and treat myself with compassion and self-love.

My self-care vision:

Once you've established your vision, you can then start to intentionally choose practices, actions, or activities that support that vision, and enable you to build up your own wellbeing and balance so you can give back to others. Use the reflection questions below to support this process.

What are the strategies that resonated for me in this book that I would like to consider for my self-care practice?

Which strategies align with my vision and could support me to flourish?

For example, if your focus is to increase your self-love and self-compassion, perhaps the strategies from the gratitude and affirmations chapters (Chapters 4 and 5) may be worth prioritising.

It's important to **integrate** your self-care plan and practices into your lifestyle to ensure that you can maintain them for the longer term. I have developed a framework that breaks down the steps to **INTEGRATE** effectively. Let's break it down.

I.N.T.E.G.R.A.T.E involves clarifying your **intention**, reflecting on your **needs**, focusing on **today**, exploring and setting **goals**, considering your **reality**, deciding on how you will **achieve** what you want, identifying the best **timing**, and **evaluating** your progress.

INTEGRATE

Intention

Needs

Today

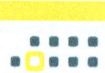

Explore

Goals

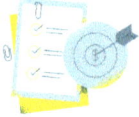

Reality

Achieve

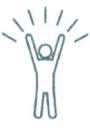

Timing

Evaluate

SOURCE: MARY MANGOS @COACHUWELLNESS

Let's I.N.T.E.G.R.A.T.E now. I recommend using the workbook or the section provided below, as you work through this framework. Revisit your reflections whenever your motivation seems to drop, and reconnect with your journal writings.

Intention

- Begin by getting clear on your intention right now. Revisit your vision and bring it to life. It is important that it becomes more than a dream and that you feel connected to it.
- Close your eyes and imagine you have achieved your vision. How do you feel? What are you doing? Where are you? Write down your thoughts and feelings.
- Now come back to the present. Set an intention for today. What do you want, right now, to be happening? Write it down.

Needs

- Reflect on what your priority needs are right now. Check in with your mind, body and spirit.
- Set your intention specifically to meet those needs.
- For example, you may have an important meeting today with your manager that you need to feel calm and focused for. Set your intention to have an amazing and successful meeting.

Today

- Now let's move your view of the day to a broader perspective.
- Consider your day and what would make it great for you today. Perhaps to end the day feeling satisfied and joyful is your broader need?
- Write that down.

Explore

- What strategies or practices are important today that will meet both your immediate and broader needs?
- Pick one practice that you wish to focus on and integrate into your lifestyle. You should feel that the practice is embedded and integrated fully before adding another.

Goals

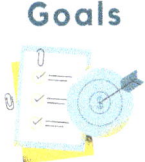

- Set a specific goal around that practice you selected. For example, 'I will meditate for 10 minutes, then I will write down one thing I am grateful for.'

Reality

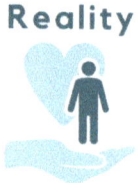

- Consider what might get in the way of your goal. For example, your kids and their immediate needs may interrupt your practice; or your phone might ring all day with calls you can't miss. Even just thinking about all the things you have to do might be a challenge to your self-care practices.

Achieve

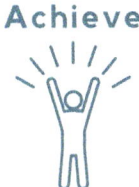

- Reflect on HOW will you achieve your goal, with full consideration of the possible blockers and challenges that may come in your day.
- How will you overcome those challenges?
- Consider if there are some lifestyle actions that you can connect your practice to. I find it can be helpful to link a practice to a daily lifestyle action. For example, when I wake up in the morning, I go to the bathroom, wash my face and then I sit and complete my morning meditation and journaling.

Timing

- Identify the best timing for you to complete the practice that supports your goal.
- Experiment and be flexible with what works best for you. Many of my clients try exercising and meditating at different times of the day when they start out, to see what they can commit to overall.
- Schedule your activity as an appointment in your calendar. Remember, this is NOT about perfection. Always be kind to yourself. If you miss a practice, there is always tomorrow.

Evaluate

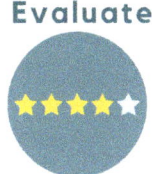

- Every week, reflect on these questions about your progress and areas for further development. Self-reflection will help you to have increased awareness of your strengths and it creates opportunities for you to develop solutions on how to adjust your actions. It can support you to achieve the goals and the self-care outcomes that you want in your life. Consider these questions:
    - When did I feel most energised?
    - When did I feel energy draining out of me?
    - What am I most grateful for?
    - What is going well?
    - What should I continue to do?
    - What do I need to do more of or do differently?

It is important to approach these reflection questions with self-compassion and kindness. If it feels challenging to answer some, then leave those and come back to them the following week. If you feel your progress is slow, remember that change can be hard. Keep in mind the reason you are doing this. Refocus back to your original desire and vision.

Inspiration for Well-*BEing* Integration

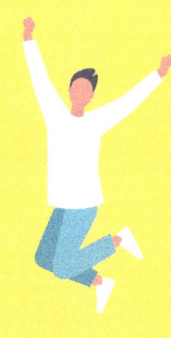

Creating a self-care plan is an important priority to support you to live well in a world full of uncertainty, high demands and stress. Self-care should be integrated into your life and feel intentional. It should be flexible according to your needs and not feel like an additional burden.

- Ensure the actions and activities you choose support your vision for *your* well-*BEing*.
- Identify the strategies in this book that align with your vision.
- Focus on today by bringing your vision into the present and then explore your thoughts and feelings.
- Check in with yourself; give yourself the space to notice any changes with your needs and to prioritise any new intentions.
- Identify what you need today. What would make it great for you right now?
- Choose practices that meet your priorities and embed them fully before considering others.
- Create specific goals to help you to break down the practice and make it feel achievable and measurable for progress.
- Identify what is happening in your world that may get in the way of your goals, so that you can understand and create solutions to overcome them.

- When you reflect on how to achieve your goals, consider your current challenges and how to build it into.
- Experiment and be flexible on the best time of day to schedule your practices.
- Do not underestimate the power of stopping to reflect and evaluate your progress. It will provide the motivation to continue on the path towards your vision and goal.
- Meditation and journaling are core practices that have contributed to my well-*BEing*, and I hope that on your well-*BEing* journey you find yours!

CHAPTER 8
Final Thoughts for Your Journey

'Life is a journey, with problems to solve and lessons to learn, but most of all, experiences to enjoy.'
Author Unknown

Over the years I have found that when I pause and reflect regularly, I will change and evolve the practices that support my well-*BEing* to ensure it continues to support my vision for peace, clarity and joy. My practices regularly shift and change as I connect with my energy and how I have been feeling, and consider what would best support my wellbeing goals. Interestingly, I have found I do have some core self-care practices that have continued during this evolution. They include:

- meditating in the morning
- journaling regularly as a way to check in with myself and what is important

- taking some time alone to enjoy my morning coffee
- lighting a candle in my office before I begin my day
- playing relaxing music while I work
- going to the gym and working for my fitness and that mental time out
- having down time outside in nature
- eating well to support my body and mind
- spending time and having fun with family and friends
- finding strategies to be able to let go of stress that arises for me during the day with breathing techniques or mindfulness
- end of the day rituals that set me up for a relaxing and peaceful evening and a great sleep.

Meditation and journaling in particular keep me on track with my wellbeing through improved self-awareness. I find that when I don't meditate in the morning I am not as focused for the rest of the day. Being organised is also important, as it supports me to continue with the practices that matter. I make space for these by scheduling and prioritising them in my day.

I have also found over time that exercising before midday is what works best for me. Even so, I find exercise is the first thing I often let go when I get busy. It is definitely something I am still working on. Right now, I won't add any more practices into my self-care plan, until I 'INTEGRATE' this one in.

Life can be challenging, but it can be amazing too. You deserve to enjoy life, so be kind to yourself. Remember it's not about perfection. This is an opportunity for you to apply your agency – your amazing capability to influence your functioning and the course of events you experience, to nourish yourself and to have a happier and healthier life.

Spending time doing and finding what well-*BEing* solutions work for you will support your wellbeing, which will have a positive influence on all those around you. Today is a new day! An opportunity for you to connect with your peace, clarity and happiness. I wish you luck and joy in the search. Please stay connected as I would love to share your journey and hear what makes a difference for you. With much love, Mary.

Acknowledgements

I would like to thank my husband Michael for always being encouraging with all of my endeavours and passions. You have always supported me, loved me, and helped me to achieve my goals and dreams. The notes and jokes that you supplied on my book draft made me smile and laugh. They kept me going forward. Lots of appreciation goes to my boys, Chris and Corey, for their love, support and letting me share our family stories.

To my Mum and Dad, thank you for your love and strength. Your example and unconditional love are what keeps me grounded and grateful always.

Dixie Maria Carlton, I am blessed to have worked with you as I developed and wrote my book. Your mentorship, friendship, feedback, and kindness will never be forgotten. I am grateful for you, and all of the Indie Experts team, for your expertise and inspiration. In particular, a special mention to Ann Dettori Wilson for connecting with me through LinkedIn and introducing me to your incredible company and services. Writing this book with you all has been the most amazing chapter of my life. I am so grateful my amazing editor Anne-Marie Tripp who took such care and interest in my words and intent. Your valuable suggestions and advice have helped to shape this book and I thank you for your work.

I am so lucky to have such amazing friends and an extended family who love and support my endeavours. They include Jola Starkowski (my dear friend who I met in my first year at university studying psychology, over 38 years ago), Dina Tselios and Jane Creasey. These three amazing women read my draft and took the time to provide valuable feedback. I also want to thank Voula Jakubicki, Mina Kondos, Kimberly Sargent and Anastasia Kourtis for reminding me I do have something valuable to share, and for their support and love.

Dr Jenny Liu, thank you for writing my foreword. I am grateful to have come across your incredible work in stress and resilience. I admire all that you do, your kindness, generosity of spirit, your mission and the inspiration you provide.

I would like to extend special thanks to a psychology educator that I admire, Dr Maria Sirois, who facilitates the Teaching for Transformation Program. Whenever self-doubt creeps in, I remember your feedback to me: 'You seem to have a gift for making things super easy to understand – this is such a talent.' Thank you, Maria!

Finally, I want to say THANK YOU to YOU. I am so incredibly joyful that you picked up my book and are reading this page. Many of you may be experiencing challenging times and situations and I believe that finding ways to bloom is possible. I believe wholeheartedly in cultivating well-*BEing* and I am so inspired by the difference that strategies from positive psychology, mindfulness and meditation have made to my life. If you are struggling with prioritising yourself, my hope is that my book will inspire you to open the door to your beautiful wellbeing journey.

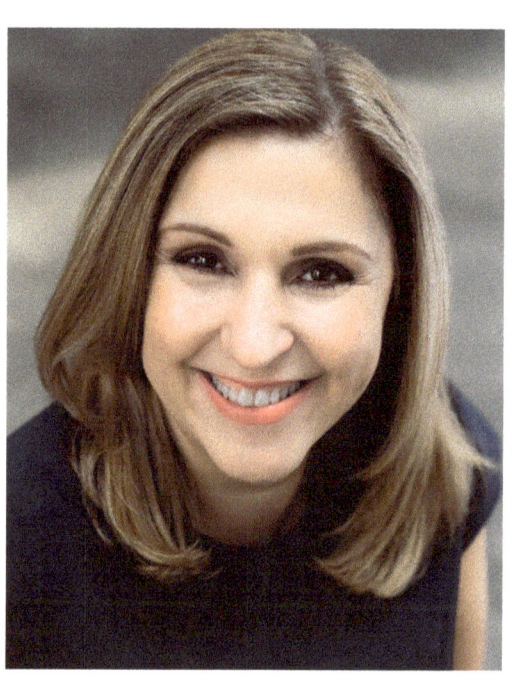

About Mary Mangos

Mary Mangos is a psychologist with over 30 years' experience, and the founder of Coachuwellness. Mary's mission has been to share positive psychology, science and wisdom that inspires individuals, teams and organisations to thrive and flourish. She has over 20 years' experience creating learning programs, leading workshops and coaching others to find calm, clarity and joy through uncertainty and change. She helps people clarify their purpose, build their resilience, reduce stress and improve their wellbeing.

Prior to creating her own business, Mary worked in human resources and organisational development roles. Some of her professional achievements include supporting Ford Australia to win the Australian Chamber of Commerce and Industry Work and Family Award, and receiving the BF Goodrich Chemical's Training Employer of the Year Award.

Her corporate clients include CEOs, executives, middle managers, team leaders and professionals. A sample of Mary's corporate clients include: Stantec, Bayer, Maxxia, Chisholm, The Women's Hospital, City of Moreland, City of Casey, City of Whitehorse and City of Kingston. She enjoys supporting everyone with the tools and strategies to achieve their wellbeing goals.

Mary regularly engages with her community on social media, sharing tips and strategies to inspire others to enhance their mental health and wellbeing. Explore more helpful ideas on Instagram through her account at https://www.instagram.com/coachuwellness/. She also has resources, including online learning, news, podcast episodes and meditations, on her website: www.coachuwellness.com.au

Mary lives in Melbourne, Australia. She is married to Michael (over 30 years), has two adult sons, Corey and Chris, and a Japanese Spitz, T.J.

Work with Mary Mangos

Mary Mangos supports professionals, teams, and organisations to flourish and thrive through uncertainty and change. If you would like to learn more about how to enhance your wellbeing, increase your calm and focus, and create your best life, please visit the Coachuwellness website at www.coachuwellness.com.au.

Here you will find a wealth of resources, including:

- the inspirational *Wellness Solutions* podcast
- accessible guided meditations for busy people
- engaging online learning programs, workshops and webinars
- information about one-on-one coaching sessions.

Mary Mangos is also a popular keynote speaker, inspiring and engaging groups on topics such as finding your well-BEing, developing emotional flexibility, and developing resilience. Mary can design keynote speeches to meet your specific needs, or as part of a broader organisational development strategies. For information on booking Mary as a keynote speaker, please email mary@coachuwellness.com.au.

Participant feedback on Mary Mangos keynote sessions:

'I really enjoyed Mary Mangos' session. I found she was engaging and it also encouraged me to engage in self-reflection. I found it to be helpful and has put me in a positive mindset and outlook for the year, which is a nice way to begin the year.'

'The keynote was very engaging and gave very practical strategies which are valuable for both professional and personal challenges.'

'I really enjoyed learning about this and Mary was very knowledgeable.'

'Fantastic; this is a very exciting and current topic amongst psychologists. Great information and great strategies. We need to do more of this kind of professional development.'

Share your journey with Mary at mary@coachuwellness.com.au, otherwise stay in touch with Mary and Coachuwellness on social media, at:

Facebook: facebook.com/coachuwellness
Twitter: twitter.com/coachuwellness
Instagram: instagram.com/coachuwellness
LinkedIn: linkedin.com/in/mary-mangos

Notes

1. Wendy Tuohy, '"I Can't Be Bothered": Victorians Battling "Compound Fatigue" of Lockdowns,' *The Age*, June 5, 2001, https://www.theage.com.au/national/victoria/i-can-t-be-bothered-victorians-battling-compounding-fatigue-of-lockdowns-20210604-p57y77.html.
2. Max Albert Holdsworth, 'La santé, le « wellness » et le bien-être,' ['Health, Wellness and Wellbeing,'] *Revue Inverventions Économiques* 62 (2019), https://doi.org/10.4000/interventionseconomiques.6322.
3. 'Wellbeing,' BetterHealth Channel, State Government of Victoria Department of Health, last modified May 27, 2020, https://www.betterhealth.vic.gov.au/health/healthyliving/wellbeing.
4. State Government of Victoria, 'Wellbeing.'
5. 'Agency,' Albert Bandura, accessed July 2, 2021, https://albertbandura.com/albert-bandura-agency.html.
6. John F. Helliwell et al., eds., *World Happiness Report 2021* (New York: Sustainable Development Solutions, 2021), 109, https://happiness-report.s3.amazonaws.com/2021/WHR+21.pdf.
7. 'Household Pulse Survey,' Centers for Disease Control and Prevention, updated August 25, 2021, https://www.cdc.gov/nchs/covid19/pulse/mental-health.htm.
8. Jane Fisher and Maggie Kirkman, *Living With COVID-19 Restrictions in Australia* (Melbourne: School of Public Health and Preventative Medicine, Monash University), accessed July 2, 2021, https://www.monash.edu/medicine/living-with-covid-19-restrictions-survey.
9. 'Mental Health: Burden,' World Health Organization, accessed July 2, 2021, https://www.who.int/health-topics/mental-health.
10. Productivity Commission, *Mental Health*, Report no. 95, (Canberra: Productivity Commission, 2020), 9, https://www.pc.gov.au/inquiries/completed/mental-health/report/mental-health-volume1.pdf.

11 'Stress,' Australian Psychological Society, accessed July 2, 2021, https://psychology.org.au/for-the-public/psychology-topics/stress
12 Tobias Esch and George B. Stefano, 'The Neurobiology of Stress Management,' *Neuroendocrinology Letters* 31, no.1 (2010): 20.
13 Carolyn Aldwin, 'Stress and Coping Across the Lifespan,' in *The Oxford Handbook of Stress, Health, and Coping*, ed. Susan Folkman (New York: Oxford University Press, 2012), 17–18.
14 'Living with Uncertainty: How to Accept and be More Comfortable with Unpredictability,' Stanford Today, Stanford University, updated November 4, 2020, https://news.stanford.edu/today/2020/11/04/living-with-uncertainty.
15 Clifford B. Saper and Bradford B. Lowell, 'The Hypothalamus,' *Current Biology* 24, no. 23 (December 2014): R1112, https://doi.org/10.1016/j.cub.2014.10.023.
16 'Understanding the Stress Response,' Harvard Medical School, updated July 6, 2020, https://www.health.harvard.edu/staying-healthy/understanding-the-stress-response; 'Stress,' Introduction to Psychology, Lumen Learning, accessed July 2, 2021, https://courses.lumenlearning.com/wmopen-psychology/chapter/introduction-defining-stress/.
17 Bruce S. McEwen, 'Stressed or Stressed Out: What is the Difference?' *Journal of Psychiatry & Neuroscience* 30, no. 5 (September 2015): 317.
18 Paul J. Lucassen et al., 'Neuropathology of Stress,' *Acta Neuropathologica* 127, no. 1 (January 2014): 109–135.
19 Kanchan Bisht, Kaushik Sharma, and Marie-Ève Tremblay, 'Chronic Stress as a Risk Factor for Alzheimer's Disease: Roles of Microglia-Mediated Synaptic Remodeling, Inflammation, And Oxidative Stress,' *Neurobiology of Stress* 9 (November 2018): 9–21, https://doi.org/10.1016/j.ynstr.2018.05.003
20 Paul H. Black, 'Stress and the Inflammatory Response: A Review of Neurogenic Inflammation,' *Brain Behavior, and Immunity* 16, no. 6 (December 2002): 622–653, https://doi.org/10.1016/S0889-1591(02)00021-1.
21 Agnese Mariotti, 'The Effects of Chronic Stress on Health: New Insights into the Molecular Mechanisms of Brain–Body Communication,' *Future Science OA* 1, no. 3, (June 2015): FSO23, https://doi.org/10.4155/fso.15.21.
22 Australian Psychological Society, 'Stress.'
23 Helliwell et al, *The World Happiness Report 2021*, 134.
24 Kristin Layous, Joseph Chancellor, and Sonja Lyubomirsky, 'Positive Activities as Protective Factors Against Mental Health Conditions,' *Journal of Abnormal Psychology* 123, no. 1 (2014): 3–12, https://doi.org/10.1037/a0034709.

25 Jenny J. W. Liu, Maureen Reed, and Todd A. Girard, 'Advancing Resilience: An Integrative, Multi-System Model of Resilience,' *Personality and Individual Differences* 111 (June 2017): 111–118, https://doi.org/10.1016/j.paid.2017.02.007.
26 Angela Lee Duckworth and Lauren Eskreis-Winkler, 'True Grit,' Association for Psychological Science, updated March 29, 2013, https://www.psychologicalscience.org/observer/true-grit.
27 Mihaly Csikszentmihalyi, *Flow: The Psychology of Optimal Experience* (New York: Harper & Row, 1990).
28 'Connect with People,' 10 Keys to Happier Living, Action for Happiness, accessed July 2, 2021, https://www.actionforhappiness.org/10-keys-to-happier-living/connect-with-people/details.
29 Susan Murphy, 'What Is Zen?' Zen Open Circle, accessed July 2, 2021, http://zenopencircle.org.au/begin/what-is-zen.
30 Natalie Goldberg, Writing Down the Bones: Freeing the Writer Within, (Colorado: Shambhala Publications, 2005), 232.
31 Steve Bradt, 'Wandering Mind Not A Happy Mind,' The Harvard Gazette, updated November 11, 2010, https://news.harvard.edu/gazette/story/2010/11/wandering-mind-not-a-happy-mind.
32 Matthew A. Killingsworth and Daniel T. Gilbert, 'A Wandering Mind is an Unhappy Mind,' *Science* 330, no. 6006 (November 2010): 932.
33 Sara W. Lazar et al., 'Meditation Experience Is Associated with Increased Cortical Thickness,' Neuroreport 16, no. 17 (November 2005): 1895, https://doi.org/10.1097/01.wnr.0000186598.66243.19.
34 These steps are inspired by Jack Kornfield, 'Practice: Don't Know Mind,' https://jackkornfield.com/practice-dont-know-mind.
35 'The Emotion Wheel: What It Is and How to Use It,' PositivePsychology.com, updated May 20, 2021, https://positivepsychology.com/emotion-wheel.
36 'National Mental Health and Wellbeing Pandemic Response Plan,' National Mental Health Commission, accessed July 2, 2021, https://www.mentalhealthcommission.gov.au/Mental-Health-and-Wellbeing-Pandemic-Response-Plan.
37 Michael D.C. Fishman, 'The Silver Linings Journal: Gratitude During A Pandemic,' *Journal of Radiology Nursing* 39, no. 3 (September 2020): 149, https://doi.org/10.1016/j.jradnu.2020.05.005.
38 Robert Emmons, 'Gratitude and Well-Being,' Gratitude Works, accessed July 2, 2021, https://emmons.faculty.ucdavis.edu/gratitude-and-well-being.
39 Fred B. Bryant and Joseph Veroff, *Savoring: A New Model of Positive Experience* (New Jersey: Lawrence Erlbaum Associates, 2007).

40 Jack Kornfield, 'Gratitude and Wonder,' accessed July 2, 2021, https://jackkornfield.com/gratitude.
41 Shauna Shapiro, *Good Morning, I Love You* (Colorado: Sounds True, 2020), 4.
42 Christopher N. Cascio et al., 'Self-affirmation Activates Brain Systems Associated with Self-Related Processing and Reward and is Reinforced by Future Orientation,' *Social Cognitive and Affective Neuroscience* 11, no. 4 (April 2016): 622, https://doi.org/10.1093/scan/nsv136.
43 David K. Sherman et al., 'Psychological Vulnerability and Stress: The Effects of Self-Affirmation on Sympathetic Nervous System Responses to Naturalistic Stressors,' *Health Psychology* 28, no. 5 (September 2009): 554–562; Clayton R. Critcher and David Dunning, 'Self-Affirmations Provide a Broader Perspective on Self-Threat,' *Personality and Social Psychology Bulletin* 41, no. 1 (January, 2015): 3–18.
44 Richard Cooke et al., 'Self-Affirmation Promotes Physical Activity,' *Journal of Sport and Exercise Psychology* 36, no. 2 (April 2014): 217–223.
45 Peter R. Harris et al., 'Self-Affirmation Reduces Smokers' Defensiveness to Graphic On-Pack Cigarette Warning Labels,' *Health Psychology* 26, no. 4 (July 2007): 437–46.
46 Tracy Epton and Peter R. Harris, 'Self-Affirmation Promotes Health Behavior Change,' *Health Psychology* 27, no. 6 (November 2008): 746–752.
47 Sander L. Koole, Ad van Knippenberg, and Ap Dijksterhuis, 'The Cessation of Rumination Through Self-Affirmation,' *Journal of Personality and Social Psychology* 77, no. 1 (1999): 111–125; Batia M. Wiesenfeld et al., 'Stress and Coping Among Layoff Survivors: A Self-Affirmation Analysis,' *Anxiety, Stress & Coping* 14, no. 1 (2001): 15–34.
48 Elaine Fox, *Rainy Brain, Sunny Brain: The New Science of Optimism and Pessimism* (London: Arrow Books, 2013): 48.
49 Kristina Fenn and Majella Byrne, 'The Key Principles of Cognitive Behavioural Therapy,' *InnovAiT* 6, no. 9 (September 2013): 579. https://doi.org/10.1177/1755738012471029.
50 'Spirituality,' VIA Institute on Character, accessed July 2, 2021, https://www.viacharacter.org/character-strengths/spirituality.
51 Christopher Peterson et al., 'Strengths of Character and Work,' in *The Oxford Handbook of Positive Psychology*, eds. Nicola Garcea, Susan Harrington, and P. Alex Linley (New York: Oxford University Press, 2010), 221–231.
52 Renzo Felipe Carranza Esteban et al., 'Spirituality and Religiousness as Predictors of Life Satisfaction Among Peruvian Citizens During the

COVID-19 Pandemic,' *Heliyon* 7, no. 5 (May 2021): e06939, https://doi.org/10.1016/j.heliyon.2021.e06939.
53 Ryan Niemiec, 'What Does Spirituality Mean to You?' VIA Institute on Character, updated April 20, 2020, https://www.viacharacter.org/topics/articles/what-does-spirituality-mean-to-you.
54 Jim Robbins, 'Ecopsychology: How Immersion in Nature Benefits Your Health,' Yale Environment 360, Yale School of the Environment, updated January 9, 2020, https://e360.yale.edu/features/ecopsychology-how-immersion-in-nature-benefits-your-health.
55 Erica H. Wise, Matthew A. Hersh, and Clare M. Gibson, 'Ethics, Self-Care and Well-Being for Psychologists: Reenvisioning the Stress-Distress Continuum,' *Professional Psychology: Research and Practice* 43, no. 5 (2012): 488; Souraya Sidani, 'Self-Care,' in *Nursing Outcomes: State of the Science*, ed. Diane Doran (Sudbury: Jones & Bartlett Learning, 2010), 81.
56 There has been a surge of interest in the concept of self-care since the 1970s, but Levin and Idler (1983), trace popular interest in self-care and self-help back to the mid-1800s, at least in the USA and other Western countries, as interest in public health reform grew, attitudes towards health and the cause of disease changed, and other social and political changes such as the changing role of women in society, were happening.
57 J. 'Jay' Miller and Erlene Grise-Owens, 'Self-Care: An Imperative,' *Social Work* 65, no. 1 (2020): 5; Nicole Spector, 'What is Self-Care? How to Cut Through the Marketing Noise and Actually Practice It,' Better, NBC News, updated February 19, 2020, https://www.nbcnews.com/better/lifestyle/what-self-care-how-cut-through-marketing-noise-actually-practice-ncna1134921.
58 Kirsten Posluns and Terry Lynn Gall, 'Dear Mental Health Practitioners, Take Care of Yourself: A Literature Review on Self-Care,' *International Journal for the Advancement of Counselling* 42, no. 1 (2020): 4.
59 These four principles are based on those suggested by Wise, Hersh and Gibson (2012) for their lifestyle changes model. While their model was developed for psychologists, the self-care strategies they suggest are useful and applicable for everyone.

Bibliography

Action for Happiness. 'Connect with People.' 10 Keys to Happier Living. Accessed July 2, 2021. https://www.actionforhappiness.org/10-keys-to-happier-living/connect-with-people/details.

Aldwin, Carolyn. 'Stress and Coping Across the Lifespan.' In *The Oxford Handbook of Stress, Health, and Coping*, edited by Susan Folkman, 15–34. New York: Oxford University Press, 2012.

Australian Psychological Society. 'Stress.' Accessed July 2, 2021. https://psychology.org.au/for-the-public/psychology-topics/stress.

Bandura, Albert. 'Agency.' Accessed July 2, 2021. https://albertbandura.com/albert-bandura-agency.html.

Bisht, Kanchan, Kaushik Sharma, Marie-Ève Tremblay. 'Chronic Stress as a Risk Factor for Alzheimer's Disease: Roles of Microglia-Mediated Synaptic Remodeling, Inflammation, And Oxidative Stress.' *Neurobiology of Stress* 9 (November 2018): 9–21. https://doi.org/10.1016/j.ynstr.2018.05.003.

Black, Paul H. 'Stress and the Inflammatory Response: A Review of Neurogenic Inflammation.' *Brain Behavior, and Immunity* 16, no. 6 (December 2002): 622–653. https://doi.org/10.1016/S0889-1591(02)00021-1.

Bouschet, Coley Lane. '50+ Intention Ideas to Set at the Start of the Year.' Life Goals Online Magazine. Accessed June 10, 2021. https://lifegoalsmag.com/50-intention-ideas-set-start-day.

Bradt, Steve. 'Wandering Mind Not A Happy Mind.' The Harvard Gazette. Updated November 11, 2010. https://news.harvard.edu/gazette/story/2010/11/wandering-mind-not-a-happy-mind.

Brenan, Megan. 'Americans' Mental Health Ratings Sink to New Low.' Gallup. Updated December 7, 2020. https://news.gallup.com/poll/327311/americans-mental-health-ratings-sink-new-low.aspx.

Breus, Michael. '7 Things to Know About the Links Between Sleep, Nutrition, and

Time.' The Sleep Doctor. Updated December 3, 2020. https://thesleepdoctor.com/2020/12/03/7-things-to-know-about-the-links-between-sleep-nutrition-and-time.

Breus, Michael. 'How to Sleep Better.' The Sleep Doctor. Accessed July 2, 2021. https://thesleepdoctor.com/how-to-sleep-better.

Brown, Joshua, and Joel Wong. 'How Gratitude Changes You and Your Brain.' Greater Good Magazine, Greater Good Science Center, University of California, Berkeley. https://greatergood.berkeley.edu/article/item/how_gratitude_changes_you_and_your_brain.

Bryant, Fred B., and Joseph Veroff. *Savoring: A New Model of Positive Experience*. New Jersey: Lawrence Erlbaum Associates, 2007.

Burton, Linda Roszak. 'The Neuroscience of Gratitude: What You Need to Know About the New Neural Knowledge.' Wharton Health Care Management Alumni Association, https://www.whartonhealthcare.org/the_neuroscience_of_gratitude.

Cascio Christopher N., Matthew Brook O'Donnell, Francis J. Tinney, Matthew D. Lieberman, Shelley E. Taylor, Victor J. Strecher, Emily B. Falk. 'Self-affirmation Activates Brain Systems Associated with Self-Related Processing and Reward and is Reinforced by Future Orientation.' *Social Cognitive and Affective Neuroscience* 11, no. 4 (April 2016): 621–629. https://doi.org/10.1093/scan/nsv136.

Centers for Disease Control and Prevention. 'Household Pulse Survey.' Updated August 25, 2021. https://www.cdc.gov/nchs/covid19/pulse/mental-health.htm.

Cooke, Richard, Helena Trebaczyk, Peter Harris, and Alison J Wright. 'Self-Affirmation Promotes Physical Activity.' *Journal of Sport and Exercise Psychology* 36, no. 2 (April 2014): 217–223.

Critcher, Clayton R., and David Dunning. 'Self-Affirmations Provide a Broader Perspective on Self-Threat.' *Personality and Social Psychology Bulletin* 41, no. 1 (January, 2015): 3–18.

Csikszentmihalyi, Mihaly. *Flow: The Psychology of Optimal Experience*. New York: Harper & Row, 1990.

Diamond, Adele. 'Executive Functions.' *Annual Review of Psychology* 64 (2013): 135–168.

Drukpa, Gyalwang. *Happiness is a State of Mind*. London: Hodder and Stoughton, 2017.

Duckworth, Angela Lee and Lauren Eskreis-Winkler. 'True Grit.' Association for Psychological Science. Updated March 29, 2013. https://www.psychologicalscience.org/observer/true-grit.

Emmons, Robert. 'Gratitude and Well-Being.' Gratitude Works. Accessed July 2, 2021. https://emmons.faculty.ucdavis.edu/gratitude-and-well-being.

Emmons, Robert. 'How Gratitude Can Help You Through Hard Times.' Greater Good Magazine, Greater Good Science Center, University of California, Berkeley. Updated May 13, 2013. https://greatergood.berkeley.edu/article/item/how_gratitude_can_help_you_through_hard_times.

Epton, Tracy, and Peter R. Harris, 'Self-Affirmation Promotes Health Behavior Change.' *Health Psychology* 27, no. 6 (November 2008): 746–752.

Esch, Tobias, and George B. Stefano. 'The Neurobiology of Stress Management.' *Neuroendocrinology Letters* 31, no.1 (2010):19–39.

Esteban, Renzo Felipe Carranza, Josue Edison Turpo-Chaparro, Oscar Mamani-Benito, Jesús Hanco Torres and Fiorella Sarria Arenaza. 'Spirituality and Religiousness as Predictors of Life Satisfaction Among Peruvian Citizens During the COVID-19 Pandemic.' *Heliyon* 7, no. 5 (May 2021): e06939. https://doi.org/10.1016/j.heliyon.2021.e06939.

Fenn, Kristina, and Majella Byrne. 'The Key Principles of Cognitive Behavioural Therapy.' *InnovAiT* 6, no. 9 (September 2013): 579–585. https://doi.org/10.1177/1755738012471029.

Fisher, Jane R. W., Thach D. Tran, Karin Hammarberg, Jayagowri Sastry, Hau Nguyen, Heather Rowe, Sally Popplestone, Ruby Stocker, Claire Stubber and Maggie Kirkman. 'Mental Health of People in Australia in the First Month of COVID-19 Restrictions: a National Survey.' *Medical Journal of Australia* 213, no. 10 (2020): 458–464. https://dx.doi.org/10.5694/mja2.50831.

Fisher, Jane, and Maggie Kirkman. *Living With COVID-19 Restrictions in Australia*. Melbourne: School of Public Health and Preventative Medicine, Monash University, 2020. Accessed July 2, 2021. https://www.monash.edu/medicine/living-with-covid-19-restrictions-survey.

Fishman, Michael D.C. 'The Silver Linings Journal: Gratitude During A Pandemic.' *Journal of Radiology Nursing* 39, no. 3 (September 2020): 149–150. https://doi.org/10.1016/j.jradnu.2020.05.005.

Fox, Elaine, *Rainy Brain, Sunny Brain: The New Science of Optimism and Pessimism*. London: Arrow Books, 2013.

Goldberg, Natalie. Writing Down the Bones: Freeing the Writer Within. Colorado: Shambhala Publications, 2005.

Greater Good Science Center, University of California, Berkeley. 'Gratitude Journal.' Greater Good in Action. Accessed June 10, 2021. https://ggia.berkeley.edu/practice/gratitude_journal?_ga=2.136931504.10651079.1596687814-1930267737.1583114207.

Greater Good Science Center, University of California, Berkeley. 'Three Good Things.' Greater Good in Action. Accessed June 10, 2021. https://ggia.berkeley.edu/practice/three-good-things?_ga=2.42016805.10651079.159668814-1930267737.1583114207.

Greater Good Science Center, University of California, Berkeley. 'Savoring Walk.' Greater Good in Action. Accessed June 10, 2021. https://ggia.berkeley.edu/practice/savoring_walk#data-tab-evidence

Grossman, Paul, Ludger Niemann, Stefan Schmidt, Harald Walach.'Mindfulness-Based Stress Reduction and Health Benefits. A Meta-Analysis.' *Journal of Psychosomatic Research* 57, no. 1 (July 2004): 35–43.

Harris, Peter R., Kathryn Mayle, Lucy Mabbott, and Lucy Napper. 'Self-Affirmation Reduces Smokers' Defensiveness to Graphic On-Pack Cigarette Warning Labels.' *Health Psychology* 26, no. 4 (July 2007): 437–46.

Harvard Medical School. 'Understanding the Stress Response.' Updated July 6, 2020. https://www.health.harvard.edu/staying-healthy/understanding-the-stress-response.

Hassed, Craig. 'The Health Benefits of Meditation and Being Mindful.' Monash University. Accessed July 2, 2021. https://www.monash.edu/__data/assets/pdf_file/0004/694192/The-health-benefits-of-meditation-and-being-mindful.pdf.

Helliwell, John F., Richard Layard, Jeffrey Sachs, and Jan-Emmanuel De Neve, eds. World Happiness Report 2021. New York: Sustainable Development Solutions Network, 2021. https://happiness-report.s3.amazonaws.com/2021/WHR+21.pdf.

Holdsworth, Max Albert, 'La santé, le « wellness » et le bien-être.' ['Health, Wellness and Wellbeing.'] Revue Inverventions Économiques 62 (2019), https://doi.org/10.4000/interventionseconomiques.6322.

Killingsworth, Matthew A., and Daniel T. Gilbert, 'A Wandering Mind is an Unhappy Mind,' *Science* 330, no. 6006 (November 2010): p. 932.

Koole, Sander L., Ad van Knippenberg, and Ap Dijksterhuis, 'The Cessation of Rumination Through Self-Affirmation." *Journal of Personality and Social Psychology* 77, no. 1 (1999): 111–125.

Kornfield, Jack. 'Gratitude and Wonder.' Accessed July 2, 2021. https://jackkornfield.com/gratitude.

Kornfield, Jack. 'Practice: Don't Know Mind.' Accessed July 2, 2021. https://jackkornfield.com/practice-dont-know-mind/

Layous, Kristin, Joseph Chancellor, and Sonja Lyubomirsky. 'Positive Activities as Protective Factors Against Mental Health Conditions.' *Journal of Abnormal Psychology* 123, no. 1 (2014): 3–12. https://doi.org/10.1037/a0034709.

Lazar Sara W., Catherine E. Kerr, Rachel H. Wasserman, Jeremy R. Gray, Douglas N. Greve, Michael T. Treadway, Metta McGarvey, Brian T. Quinn, Jeffery A. Dusek, Herbert Benson, Scott L. Rauch, Christopher I. Moore, and Bruce Fischl. 'Meditation Experience Is Associated with Increased Cortical Thickness.' Neuroreport 16, no. 17 (November 2005): 1893–1897. https://doi.org/10.1097/01.wnr.0000186598.66243.19.

Levin, Lowell S. and Ellen L. Idler. 'Self-Care in Health.' *Annual Review of Public Health* 4 (1983): 181–201.

Liu, Jenny J. W., Maureen Reed, and Todd A. Girard. 'Advancing Resilience: An Integrative, Multi-System Model of Resilience.' *Personality and Individual Differences* 111 (June 2017): 111–118. https://doi.org/10.1016/j.paid.2017.02.007.

Lucassen, Paul J., Jens Preussner, Nuno Sousa, Osborne F. X. Almeida, Anne Marie Van Dam, Grazyna Rajkowska, Dick F. Swaab, and Boldizsár Czéh. 'Neuropathology of Stress.' *Acta Neuropathologica* 127, no. 1 (January 2014): 109–135.

Lumen Learning. 'Stress.' Introduction to Psychology. Accessed July 2, 2021. https://courses.lumenlearning.com/wmopen-psychology/chapter/introduction-defining-stress/.

Mariotti, Agnese. 'The Effects of Chronic Stress on Health: New Insights into the Molecular Mechanisms of Brain–Body Communication.' *Future Science OA* 1, no. 3, (June 2015): FSO23. https://doi.org/10.4155/fso.15.21.

McEwen, Bruce S. 'Stressed or Stressed Out: What is the Difference?' *Journal of Psychiatry & Neuroscience* 30, no. 5 (September 2015): 315–318.

Miller, J. 'Jay', and Erlene Grise-Owens. 'Self-Care: An Imperative.' *Social Work* 65, no. 1 (2020): 5–9.

Murphy, Susan. 'What Is Zen?' Zen Open Circle. Accessed July 2, 2021. http://zenopencircle.org.au/begin/what-is-zen.

National Mental Health Commission. 'National Mental Health and Wellbeing Pandemic Response Plan.' Accessed July 2, 2021. https://www.mentalhealthcommission.gov.au/Mental-Health-and-Wellbeing-Pandemic-Response-Plan.

Niemiec, Ryan. 'What Does Spirituality Mean to You?' VIA Institute on Character. Updated April 20, 2020. https://www.viacharacter.org/topics/articles/what-does-spirituality-mean-to-you.

Peterson, Christopher, John Paul Stephens, Nansook Park, Fiona Lee, and Martin E.P. Seligman. 'Strengths of Character and Work.' In *The Oxford Handbook of Positive Psychology*, edited by Nicola Garcea, Susan Harrington, and P. Alex Linley, 221–231. New York: Oxford University Press, 2010.

PositivePsychology.com. 'The Emotion Wheel: What It Is and How to Use It.' Updated May 20, 2021. https://positivepsychology.com/emotion-wheel.

Posluns, Kirsten and Terry Lynn Gall. 'Dear Mental Health Practitioners, Take Care of Yourself: A Literature Review on Self-Care.' *International Journal for the Advancement of Counselling* 42, no. 1 (2020): 1–20.

Productivity Commission. *Mental Health*. Report no. 95. Canberra: Productivity Commission, 2020). https://www.pc.gov.au/inquiries/completed/mental-health/report/mental-health-volume1.pdf.

Robbins, Jim. 'Ecopsychology: How Immersion in Nature Benefits Your Health.' Yale Environment 360, Yale School of the Environment. Updated January 9, 2020. https://e360.yale.edu/features/ecopsychology-how-immersion-in-nature-benefits-your-health.

Royal Melbourne Hospital. 'Connect.' 5 Ways to Wellbeing. Accessed July 2, 2021. https://5waystowellbeing.org.au/5-ways/connect/.

Saper, Clifford B., and Bradford B. Lowell. 'The Hypothalamus.' *Current Biology* 24, no. 23 (December 2014): R1111-R1116. https://doi.org/10.1016/j.cub.2014.10.023.

Shapiro, Shauna. *Good Morning, I Love You*. Colorado: Sounds True, 2020.

Sherman, David K., Debra P. Bunyan, J. David Creswell, and Lisa M. Jaremka. 'Psychological Vulnerability and Stress: The Effects of Self-Affirmation on Sympathetic Nervous System Responses to Naturalistic Stressors.' *Health Psychology* 28, no. 5 (September 2009): 554–562.

Sidani, Souraya. 'Self-Care.' in *Nursing Outcomes: State of the Science*, edited by Diane Doran, 79–124. Sudbury: Jones & Bartlett Learning, 2010.

Spector, Nicole. 'What is Self-Care? How to Cut Through the Marketing Noise and Actually Practice It.' Better, NBC News. Updated February 19, 2020. https://www.nbcnews.com/better/lifestyle/what-self-care-how-cut-through-marketing-noise-actually-practice-ncna1134921.

Stanford University, Stanford School of Medicine. 'Setting an Intention.' Updated August 12, 2015. https://mindful.stanford.edu/2015/08/setting-an-intention.

Stanford University. 'Living with Uncertainty: How to Accept and be More Comfortable with Unpredictability.' Stanford Today. Updated November 4, 2020. https://news.stanford.edu/today/2020/11/04/living-with-uncertainty.

State Government of Victoria Department of Health. 'Wellbeing.' Better Health Channel. Updated May 27, 2020. https://www.betterhealth.vic.gov.au/health/healthyliving/wellbeing.

Tuohy, Wendy. '"I Can't Be Bothered": Victorians Battling "Compound Fatigue" of Lockdowns.' *The Age*, June 5, 2001. https://www.theage.com.au/national/victoria/i-can-t-be-bothered-victorians-battling-compounding-fatigue-of-lockdowns-20210604-p57y77.html.

Van Beusekom, Mary. 'Depression Triples in US Adults Amid COVID-19 Stressors.' Center for Infectious Disease Research and Policy, University of Minnesota. Updated September 3, 2020. https://www.cidrap.umn.edu/news-perspective/2020/09/depression-triples-us-adults-amid-covid-19-stressors

VIA Institute on Character. 'Spirituality.' Accessed July 2, 2021. https://www.viacharacter.org/character-strengths/spirituality.

Wei, Allen. '8 Mindfulness Habits You Can Practice Everyday.' Project Happiness. Accessed July 2, 2021. https://shop.projecthappiness.org/blogs/project-happiness/8-mindfulness-habits-you-can-practice-everyday.

Weill Institute for Neurosciences. 'Executive Functions.' Accessed July 2, 2021. https://memory.ucsf.edu/symptoms/executive-functions.

Wiesenfeld, Batia M., Joel Brockner, Barbara Petzall, Richard Wolf and James Bailey. 'Stress and Coping Among Layoff Survivors: A Self-Affirmation Analysis.' *Anxiety, Stress & Coping* 14, no. 1 (2001): 15–34.

Wise, Erica H., Matthew A. Hersh, and Clare M. Gibson. 'Ethics, Self-Care and Well-Being for Psychologists: Re-envisioning the Stress-Destress Continuum.' *Professional Psychology Research and Practice* 43, no. 5 (January 2012): 487–494.

World Health Organization. 'Mental Health: Burden.' Accessed July 2, 2021. https://www.who.int/health-topics/mental-health.

www.ingramcontent.com/pod-product-compliance
Lightning Source LLC
Chambersburg PA
CBHW051537010526
44107CB00064B/2763